The Excellence Model in the Health Sector
Sharing good practice

First Published 2000
KINGSHAM Press
Oldbury Complex
Marsh Lane
Easthampnett, Chichester
West Sussex PO18 OJW
U.K

(c) 2000   Henry Stahr, Brenda Bulman, Michael Stead

Typeset in Garamond

Printed and Bound by MPG Books
Bodmin
Cornwall U.K

ISBN: **0-9527912-5 -0**

British Library Cataloguing in Publication Data
A catalogue record of this book is available from the British Library
Stahr, H; Bulman, B; Stead, M.

The Excellence Model in the Health Sector
Sharing good practice

edited by

Henry Stahr: Excellence Development Manager, Salford Royal Hospitals NHS Trust & Director of the Centre for Excellence Development; NHS Learning Centre, University of Salford, UK.

Brenda Bulman: Senior Quality and Organisational Development Advisor, South Tees Acute Hospitals NHS Trust, Middlesbrough, UK.

and

Michael Stead: Formerly Director of Quality, Evaluation and Development at Wakefield & Pontefract Community Health NHS Trust; now Continuous Improvement Manager at the Nuffield Hospital (Northern Division), Harrogate, UK.

KINGSHAM

List of Contributors

Case Study 1

Henry Stahr

has a dual role as Excellence Development Director at Salford Royal Hospitals NHS Trust and Director of the Centre for Excellence Development and the NHS Learning Centre at the University of Salford. Henry has a BA (Hons) in Psychology, an MSc in Management and has just completed a PhD on Heuristics and Soft Systems of Health Care Risk Management.

Case Study 2

Brenda Bulman

is Senior Quality and Organisational Development Advisor at South Tees Acute Hospitals NHS Trust. Brenda was originally a midwife and has a post-graduate Diploma in Health Services Management and an MA in Leading Innovation and Change from the University of York.

Maxine Connor

is Director of the Northern and Yorkshire Learning Alliance which delivers the South Tees Acute Hospitals National Learning contract, provides Service Improvement support and Learning for the Northern and Yorkshire Region and Consultancy support to the NHS. Maxine has a BA in Nursing and Research and an MSc in Organisational Change and Management Development.

Case Study 3

Michael Stead

was the Head of Quality, Evaluation and Development at Wakefield and Pontefract Community Health NHS Trust. He is now Continuous Improvement Manager for the Nuffield Hospitals (Northern Division). Mike has an MSc in Organisational Psychology from the University of Sheffield and an MBA from Durham University Business School.

Sharon Fennell

is Health Informatics Development Manager at Wakefield and Pontefract Community Health NHS Trust. She gained a BA(Hons) in Speech and Language Therapy at the University of Reading and an MA in Management and Leadership at the Nuffield Institute for Health at the University of Leeds.

Acknowledgements

The book is a testament to the efforts, support and hard work of a large number of staff and individuals from the three organisations. Their collective efforts have been instrumental at achieving significant improvements through the use of the Excellence Model. We are grateful to them all.

At Salford, we wish to express our thanks to Mr Peter Mount, the Chairman of Salford Royal Hospitals Trust, who first introduced the Trust to the ideas contained within the EFQM Model and to Mr William Sang, Chief Executive, whose leadership made it possible to turn theory into practice.

A number of individuals at the Wakefield & Pontefract Community Health NHS Trust, have been directly helpful in the writing of the case study and we gratefully acknowledge their help and support. In particular, we would like to extend our warm appreciation of the support and co-operation of Ray Wilk, the Chief Executive of the Trust, Hazel Walshaw, Director of Nursing and Corporate Development and Ian Bateman, the Strategic Planning Manager.

At South Tees Acute Hospitals NHS Trust, we extend a big thank you to the Chief Executive, Bill Murray and to Trish Stokoe for their contributions and support. A number of other colleagues would recognise the part their own reports and documents have played at informing and shaping this case study, and we are grateful to them for such help. Maxine Connor has played a far greater role than that of co-author, and has provided invaluable support throughout.

Contents

Preface

Preface

The Excellence Model in the health sector

The European Foundation for Quality Management (EFQM) Excellence Model is attracting considerable interest across all sectors in the United Kingdom. Since its introduction in 1991, it has become one of the most recognised frameworks for promoting excellence in organisations, large and small, private and public sector alike. The Model is regarded as a management tool which provides effective strategic and practical approaches, to enable organisations to develop excellence. It provides the means by which organisations can assess their path and develop solutions to achieve excellence.

The Model was initially adopted in the industrial and manufacturing sectors. Adoption in the public and voluntary sector took some time, with early adopters in health, education and local government coming on stream during the mid 90s.

Several initiatives, most notably those by the Cabinet Office have been established to promote the use of the Model in the health care sector. The NHS Executive has provided a central lead in endorsing the Model as an important and useful framework for delievering on the Clinical Governance agenda and the British Association of Medical Managers (BAMM), has promoted its use as a tool for organisational SELF ASSESSMENT. Recently, the NHS Alliance has added support for the Model in Primary Care Organisations, through its regional development programme. In addition, the British Quality Foundation (BQF) as guardians and promoters of the Model in the United Kingdom, continue to provide a major educational and support role on the use and adoption of the model, in health care and all other sectors across the corporate landscape.

At institutional level, more and more health care organisations are now making use of specialist support through the NHS Learning Centres and Regional networks. In addition, a number are making direct investment in getting key staff members through Excellence Model 'Assessor' training programmes, as a means of developing expertise and practical hands on experiences, towards adoption. Some are investing considerable amounts of resources at a range of 'in-house' training and development activities, in order to ensure that those at the forefront of implementing and using the Model, are adequately prepared for their roles. Equally important is the culture of learning from others and the sharing of good practice, advanced through networking, visits, secondments, Learning Networks, Resource Centres, and related publications.

This book deals with the journey through adoption and the experiences gained by three health care organisations. As early adopters of the Excellence Model, they have become the vital few at the leading edge of implementation and as such have a great deal to share and reflect upon. Their case studies provide detailed accounts on:

- why was the Model adopted?
- who were the drivers behind adoption?
- how was adoption initiated, sustained and fully implemented?

- what was achieved?
- what lessons have been learnt?

The accounts provide a wealth of insights on the stages through adoption, and experiences derived from the different applications of the Model. They vary in style, approach and focus. Each account shares a number of common features though. They reflect on the respective organisational contexts, reasons for adopting the Model and of the manner and means by which implementation was approached. The case studies are a testament to the achievements of these three organisations and the account here is seen as a contribution to the sharing of good practice, which is a vital mechanism for learning within the NHS.

Many health care staff will be familiar with the Model through a variety of sources, including Excellence Model Assessor Training, EFQM and BQF publications, workshops and conferences. The case studies are however structured in such a manner that those less familiar with the model would still be able to gain a great deal from the accounts provided here. This preface serves both to introduce the case studies as well as provide an overview of the Excellence Model. In some cases, the overview will serve as a refresher on the key premises of the Model.

Background to the EFQM Excellence Model.

The need for the development of strategic capability in the corporate world has been one of the most dominant themes from leading management commentators over recent decades. Pragmatically, many organisations have responded to this through the adoption of well tested management frameworks, models and systems. The Malcolm Baldrige National Quality Award (MBNQA) as promoted by the federal government in the United States is a case in point.

Europe was quick to realise the value of such a framework and in September 1988, the presidents of 14 leading Western European companies, signed a letter of intent to establish the European Foundation for Quality Management (EFQM). The letter was prefaced by the then President of the European Commission, Jacques Delors, who commented that:
"the battle for quality is one of the prerequisites for the success of your companies and of your collective success".

The Foundation was established in October 1989, with the remit to promote business excellence and Total Quality Management (TQM) in Europe, as well as enhancing the competitive position of European Companies through quality improvement efforts. The European Quality Award (EQA) evolved from the European Model for TQM and was influenced by the MBQNA. It was launched in October 1991 and became known in 1996 as the EFQM Business Excellence Model. Since then, a number of major companies have won the Award based on the Model which was one of the first frameworks to emphasise business results. Moreover, EQA winners had to demonstrate that they had contributed to satisfying the expectations of their customers, employees and other stakeholders. The

Model was pre-eminent at integrating TQM as a mainstream business activity. In 1992, The British Quality Foundation (BQF) was established with the aim of enhancing the performance and effectiveness of organisations in the UK, through the use of proven quality techniques as well as to promote and support the use of the Model. In 1999, the EFQM Excellence Model was revised in order to make it more attractive to public and voluntary sector companies.

The EFQM Excellence Model

The key premise of the Model is that *excellent results with respect to Performance, Customers, People and Society are achieved through Leadership driving Policy and Strategy, People, Partnerships and Resources, and Processes.* The key elements/criteria are schematically outlined below.

The EFQM Excellence Model

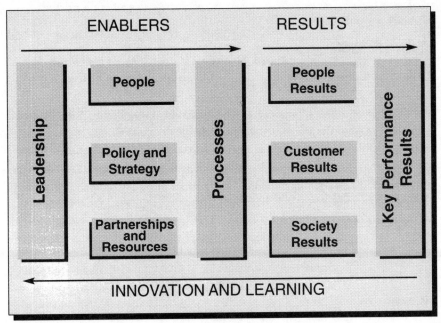

©1999 EFQM The Model is a registered trade mark of the EFQM

As is the case of the Malcolm Baldrige Award, a certain number of percentage points are assigned to each of the nine elements/criteria of the Excellence Model, reflecting their relative importance to the achievement of excellence. The Model is split 50-50 between *enablers* and *results. Enablers* are concerned with how the organisation approaches each of the areas identified. Each enabler criterion is broken down into a number of parts, which in turn are supplemented by a list of *areas to address.* Though self assessment processes, organisations are required to assess the excellence of the approach used and the extent of the deployment of each approach at all levels, areas and activities. The results criteria are concerned with what the organisation has achieved and is achieving. They are to be assessed in terms of the organisation's actual performance, its own targets and where possible, the performance of competitors and that of 'best in class' organisations.

The key criteria of the Excellence Model.

- *Leadership*
  -How leaders develop and facilitate the achievement of the mission and vision, develop values required for long term success and implement these via appropriate actions and behaviours, and the extent to which they are personally involved in ensuring that the organisation's management system is developed and implemented.

- *People*
  - How the organisation manages, develops and releases the knowledge and full potential of its people at an individual, team based and organisation-wide level, and plans these activities in order to support its policy and strategy and the effective operation of its processes.

- *Policy & Strategy*
  -How the organisation implements its mission and vision via a clear stakeholder focused strategy, supported by relevant policies, plans, objectives, targets and processes.

- *Partnerships & Resources*
  -How the organisation plans and manages its external partnerships and internal resources in order to support its policy and strategy and the effective operation of its processes.

- *Processes*
  - How the organisation designs, manages and improves its processes in order to support its policy and strategy and fully satisfy, and generate increasing value for its customers and other stakeholders.

- *People Results*
  -What the organisation is achieving in relation to its people.

- *Customer Results*
  -What the organisation is achieving in relation to its external customers.

- *Society Results*
  -What the organisation is achieving in relation to local, national and international society as appropriate.

- *Key Performance Results*
  -What the organisation is achieving in relation to its planned performance.

(Source BQF)

The manner in which these elements and criteria operate will be made evident through the substance and account of experiences discussed in the case studies.

Case Study 1
Salford Royal Hospitals
NHS Trust

1.1 Introduction

When I am asked to speak about the use of the European Foundation for Quality Management (EFQM) Model at Salford Royal Hospitals, three questions commonly recur. They are :

- *when did you introduce it?*
- *how long did it take?*
- *did it work?*

On the face of it, these are simple questions that require a straight forward answer. However, in attempting to answer these questions, it becomes clear that a useful and straight forward answer is not at as easy as one may think.

Take for example the question, 'when did you introduce it?' There are so many ways of interpreting this simple query and the answer could in effect have several starting points. It could for instance refer to the moment when I was introduced to the Model by the Trust's new Chairman, or to the time when a couple of us had our initial training. But it could also refer to the occasion when the senior management team decided to use it as a management tool. Perhaps more pragmatically, it could refer to the time when I started the process of convincing others that it should be used, or when the Trust Board formally approved it, or to the date when the top management team started to use it and when it became integrated into the Trust's management arrangements. A simple straight forward answer is therefore rather difficult and in fairness, it is not possible to give a 'start date' because the EFQM process is an enhancement of good management practice. It is part of the continual improvement of that practice, that has several starting points.

The second question 'how long did it take' is equally problematic, for it assumes that there is a point at which using the EFQM Excellence Model is completed. However, there can be no such point as the Model is a tool for diagnosing the current health of an organisation. And like all quality tools it is never completely used, because what it is used for and how effectively it is used grows with the skills of those who use it. What is completed, is that which you create using the tool. Some use it to gain recognition through submitting a self-assessment for a regional, national or European award. Others use it to set an overall strategy by identifying strengths and areas for improvement. And others use it as a way through which they can understand a particular problem which they wish to solve.

Salford chose to use the EFQM Excellence Model to provide a framework by which it could continually improve its approaches to clinical and non-clinical management. And since there is no point at which continual improvement ends, there is correspondingly no point at which the approach is complete.

The final question '*did it work?*' can be made more apt by rephrasing it to '*does it work?*' However, this question misses the point of a quality tool. A quality tool is vital if you are to create something worthwhile, but a tool is only a tool. To create something worthwhile with a quality tool depends on the vision, knowledge, skills, talent and motivation of those who use it.

 At the outset then, it is therefore important to point out that there are several layers from which one can reflect upon one's experience. My intention is to provide an account which embodies some of the fundamental ideas behind the concept of 'reflection in practice', which is now well embedded in context of vocational education in health, management and other professions. The approach that I would use draws on the work of Schon (1987), in which reflection is the basis from which insight and knowledge can be derived from our observations of concrete experience of practice or action. I would tell it as it is, but I would also pose questions, in order to generate thinking and testing of ideas based on the use of the EFQM Model.

In this case study, I will therefore reflect upon and share on Salford Royal Hospitals experience of using the EFQM Model, as a framework for achieving its mission. In order to achieve this, I will:-

- *explain how we discovered the EFQM Excellence Model,*
- *why we became interested in using it,*
- *what it is useful for and*
- *how it complements other tools needed to achieve our mission.*

I will also *share our successes and failures* in the use of the Model in order to help others not to make the same mistakes. Hopefully, this may provide some key lessons for future users of the Model who are embarking on its use, in order to achieve their own mission of continuous improvement. First though, some background and contextual details on our organisation is warranted.

1.2 Salford Royal Hospitals NHS Trust

Salford Royal Hospitals NHS Trust is a large inner city teaching hospital. The Hospital was opened on 19th October, 1882 by the Salford Board of Guardians as a Poor Law Infirmary in order to relieve overcrowding in the local workhouse. In 1925, it became a hospital for general treatment carrying out about 500 operations and delivering 366 births in that year. During the 1930's, the hospital continued to grow with the addition of outpatient and consultant specialities. On 5th July 1948, the hospital became part of the National Health Service. It continued to grow and in 1974, became a teaching hospital of the University of Manchester Medical School.

Salford Royal Hospitals NHS Trust now provides comprehensive adult general and specialist hospital services to the people of Salford. The Trust has a budget of around £100,000,000 per year and employs about 3,400 staff. It is also one of the three teaching hospitals associated with the University of Manchester Faculty of Medicine, Dentistry and Nursing. It is involved in significant research and teaching activities. Its primary focus is to provide treatment and care for approximately 70,000 A&E patient visits, 200,000 outpatient attendance and 47,000 inpatients per year. In addition, it provides a number of specialist services such as Neuroscience, Renal, Intestinal Failure and Neonatal Intensive Care for Greater Manchester, the Northwest region and the rest of the United Kingdom.

1.3 The Pursuit of Excellence prior to the discovery of the EFQM Excellence Model

It can be argued that Salford Royal Hospitals NHS Trust started its pursuit of excellence when it was first founded in 1882, and it had been very successful in this pursuit because by the time I had arrived in 1989, the Trust already had a high standing as a clinical, academic and research centre. However, there was a feeling that management was not as focused on clinical quality. A Resource Management team which had been established to bring clinicians into management and introduce the use of technology to provide meaningful, timely and comprehensive information for decision making decided to adopt Total Quality Management (TQM), as the approach for placing quality at the Centre of both clinical and managerial processes.

In 1993, the year preceding the establishment of the Trust as a legal entity in April 1994, the Resource Management team had developed and articulated its approach to quality management. It built on what the team had learnt from audit, TQM, Resource Management Initiative and existing structures so that quality development and day to day management would be totally integrated. The approach acknowledged that the patient's experience and the outcome of hospital treatment, usually involves numerous contributions from different specialities and professions that needed to be welded together into a unified high quality integrated service. The planned approach built on six foundation 'stones'. These are:

audit or quality cycle - plan, do, check, review

clarity of purpose

management action

sound information

teamwork

organisational learning (no re-inventing the wheel).

The quality cycle was to be the hub of the management system. It had to be the key method of setting, maintaining, adjusting and improving standards of service. For this to be effective, there had to be management action, reliable information and effective problem solving.

Clarity of the common purpose was considered to be a key element of success. Without clear service objectives, much energy would be consumed unproductively. The process had to extend seamlessly from the strategic hospital objectives, to detailed individual patient treatment plans.

Quality management was to be the management process because quality management implied inexorable, incremental change for the better, i.e. continuous quality improvement. It is axiomatic that the entire management process must adopt the philosophy and practice comprehensively. The aim of the approach to quality is described below and the aim was to implement this at Clinical Management Team, Directorate, Executive Board and Trust Board level.

At that time the belief was that success was dependent on:

- *good, timely, appropriate and accurate information on performance.*

- *teamwork, embodying the value of true multi-professional collaboration.*

- *problem solving through the application of quality management tools and techniques.*

- *management action for empowering the teams to bring about change.*

- *sharing of successful solutions which were widely understood and adopted throughout the organisation in order to prevent wasteful duplication of effort.*

- *developing a culture of quality so that all of this was not seen as extra work, but one in which work was carried out effectively and efficiently.*

When trying to introduce these changes, it became clear there were a number of fundamental factors which made such change difficult. The first was that the traditional management systems described a hierarchical relationship. Senior staff were employed in the organisation in terms of authority, roles and responsibilities. Such descriptions were essential, if staff were to work co-operatively with each other and focus their activities on that which is important to the organisation as a whole.

However, hierarchical management systems also have fundamental weaknesses. Their focus tends to be on who has authority and responsibility over whom within discrete management domains such as departments, professional and speciality groups. But patient care and treatment is a process which rarely falls exclusively within any single management domain. A patient, for example, may need diagnostic services from both pathology and radiology; treatment from different speciality doctors, nurses, physiotherapists and occupational therapists who in turn may need equipment and facilities maintained by medical physics and site management. Traditional management systems with their focus on top down and bottom up processes, tended to neglect the horizontal processes which the patient experiences. Furthermore, these horizontal processes tend not to be managed as efforts and are compartmentalised within functions or departments. The result is a loss of efficiency for the organisation as a whole, wasteful use of resources, extra work and frustration for staff. Importantly, it causes poor services to the patient.

The second problem was that of defining quality. The Trust therefore defined quality as *"meeting the agreed requirements of those for whom the service is provided"*. We had a broad understanding that this would include quality for external clients, such as patients and general practitioners and internal clients such as work colleagues.

Patients judge quality from their personal experience of service and the personal outcomes of treatment. Purchasers judge quality in terms of health gain for the population and value for money. Providers judge quality in terms of professional requirements and standards. There can be agreement on what quality is from each perspective, and for example, 'patients should not develop pressure sores', is a case in point. However, there can also be areas in which quality varies from one perspective to another. For instance, the patient wants to be seen at the agreed appointment time and have as much time with the doctor as they feel they need. Purchasers may require as many patients as possible to be seen, so that resources are economically used. The doctor may want to concentrate on the clinically critical conditions, whilst some clinical researchers may want to concentrate on rare and interesting conditions. Achieving quality for one person may mean compromising quality for someone else and we did not have a mechanism for dealing with this.

We also found that there was no clear and shared vision of the desired "quality state". Staff tended to focus on delivering the service but did not have a systematic way of capturing their customers requirements or assessing how effectively staff were delivering those requirements. They also did not have the skills to critically analyse the work they performed, in order that poor processes could be removed and waste and rework eliminated. Senior staff and managers generally did not provide clear objectives or facilitated the use of improvement tools and techniques, and there was little coaching and support for staff teams to help them ensure necessary change was implemented.

In sum, there was no overall framework which supported the development of quality management activities amongst all staff. More critically, there was especially nothing to help:

ensure that the whole organisation's efforts were focused on the requirements of its customers particularly patients, general practitioners and purchasers.

break down barriers between staff by promoting the recognition of the value of each person's role in achieving continual quality improvement.

clarify the relationship between various organisational structures and their processes so as to optimise their effectiveness in continually improving quality.

bind all activities together in order to facilitate and co-ordinate the quality promoting activities of the whole organisation.

ensure that learning took place across the organisation.

1.4 Health Care Quality Management (HCQM) Framework (1993)

In order to address some of these fundamental shortcomings, the organisation committed itself to a quality framework. At this time, the General Hospitals Unit as Salford Royal Hospitals was previously named, was preparing itself to become a self-managed Trust. Continuous quality improvement was to be the primary focus of the new Trust's activities and this was clearly stated in the its mission statement:

'Continually pursue clinical, academic and service excellence'.

The intention was for the Management Board to turn the Trust Board's vision into reality by ensuring that organisational systems and people were capable of achieving the strategic and operational objectives set by the Trust Board. This was to be done through the line management structure, which would have a strong clinical leadership element, through the establishment of clinical directorates.

Not being aware of the European Foundation for Quality Management (EFQM) Framework which was developed in industry in 1988, the Trust attempted to develop its own overall framework for clinical and non-clinical management within the Trust. That framework the Trust named **Health Care Quality Management (HCQM)**.

Within this HCQM framework, the Executive Medical Director was to take the lead role on the Management Board for ensuring, on behalf of the Chief Executive and Trust Board, that the functional divisions of the organisation were co-ordinated and were targeted on the Trust Board's strategic quality objectives. The Executive Medical Director was to ensure that quality performance was monitored against the Trust Board's standards and targets, good practice was identified and shared across the hospital and barriers impeding the optimal functioning of processes, were identified and removed. His primary functions were to include:

assisting the Board to integrate quality into its business strategy by ensuring that quality issues were represented in all strategic decisions.

assisting the Board to set key quality performance objectives which were focused on and responsive to the needs of the hospital's customers, particularly patients, general practitioners and purchasers.

ensuring that corporate quality review was carried out, quality performance reports are produced and published and a strategy for risk management developed.

identifying common themes and problems which needed action and bringing these to the attention of the appropriate manager or clinician.

ensuring the implementation of agreed quality policies and procedures.

co-ordinating the application of Quality Management processes in order to optimise the functioning of the whole organisation

promoting and ensuring the sharing of good practice across the hospital, including providing facilitation to the Board and Directorates in the application of quality management techniques.

ensuring research into clinical and non-clinical quality management is carried out and appropriate findings implemented.

In order to assist the Executive Medical Director to carry out these functions, a Trust HCQM Team was established. The membership of this team included the Executive Medical Director (Chair), Chief Executive, Hospital Lead Clinician (Audit), Corporate Quality Manager, General Managers, Marketing and Contracting Director, Executive Nurse and Director of Facilities.

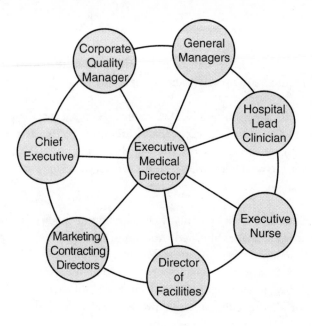

This team was to ensure that systematic attention was paid to horizontal linkage and integration across the organisation. In addition, it had to ensure that the processes delivering care and other outputs, were optimised in line with the Hospital's Corporate Quality Objectives. The Team's functions were to:

- assist the Executive Medical Director in carrying out the key functions listed above.
- provide specialist advice on quality matters to the Board and others as required.
- facilitate the development of staff within clinical management teams so that they were capable of carrying out their function within the Quality System.
- ensure the sharing of good practice across the whole organisation.
- provide support to Facilitators, Quality Development Teams (QDT's) and Audit Leaders.
- keep staff informed of developments in Quality
- identify common educational and training deficiencies and implementing appropriate training programmes
- identify the best methods to measure clinical and non-clinical quality performance in such a way that it was accurate, timely, meaningful and useful in decision making and marketing.
- identify key horizontal processes which were critical for organisational success.

- develop key system management processes which were consistent with the HCQM approach.
- develop corporate quality standards which are sensitive to patient and purchaser requirements and within the capability of the Unit to deliver.

Establishing a fully functioning HCQM system was not expected to develop quickly. Not only would the structures and functions required take time to implement, but there was also a great deal of education and training required, if all staff were to have the knowledge and skills required to work effectively within the system.

However, it was recognised that many areas of good quality management practice were already well established. Audit and quality development teams were already functioning in many areas. Directorate quality performance was being developed in several speciality areas by their own quality assurance boards and quality development teams. Monitoring of quality performance with links to contracting and marketing processes were also well developed.

However, a great deal of management practice can best be described as fire fighting and it was difficult to assess whether the Trust had improved, remained the same or had deteriorated in any of the key dimensions of its mission. Only finance and activity, were systematically measured but these two measures had little credence with the clinical staff or patients. Fundamentally, the basic process of any quality system is a feedback loop, but a well structured regular feedback loop did not exist within the Trust.

1.5 The Discovery of the European Foundation for Quality Management (EFQM) Model 1994.

In April, 1994 the first Chairman of the Trust was appointed together with the Trust's Chief Executive. The Chief Executive had been fully supportive of the quality management approach developed prior to the Trust being formed, and attended and supported the training and awareness raising activities developed to promote continuous improvement. However, our Chairman had previous experience of using the EFQM Model in industry and he suggested that we needed to adopt a well tried and tested Model, in order to give a firmer structure to our approach to HCQM. The Chairman maintained that the EFQM approach would also provide the much needed comprehensive performance feedback loop we needed, in order to measure progress and identify our strengths and areas for improvement.

Our initial idea at the time was to use the Model to energise our quality management strategy by giving us the target of achieving the European Quality Award by 1996, a target set by the Chairman in his maiden speech to the Trust's staff. On reflection, I don't think that either of us believed we could win, but that was not the point. The idea was that the challenge would give focus to the quality management effort.

The immediate problem was to gain some expertise in EFQM. Following discussion with a colleague at the University of Salford, a mutual need was met by offering a PhD studentship, to pursue an action research based study within the Trust. This was seen as vital to support my responsibility to introduce the EFQM process into the Trust.

The PhD student and I both undertook training in EFQM provided by a Consultancy Firm and both became licensed assessors in November, 1994. It was clear from this training that the approach taught by this company would not be a practical way forward within our organisation which had serious financial constraints on its training budget. More importantly, it was also ambitious on the demand on time that people would be able to make available for training. We therefore developed a plan, based on some of the insights gained during the implementation of the TQM approach, prior to 1994.

1.6　Top down and integrated approach

We decided to start at the top and not to attempt to work bottom up, as was the case when we introduced TQM. The reason for this was that with insufficient resources, it would be impossible to adequately support a bottom-up effort, especially when it hit problems. In addition, one key reason why our previous bottom-up approach ran into difficulties, was that some line managers felt threatened by an approach which they did not fully understood themselves. More critical though, was the fact that middle management's opposition increased when they felt that the effort required to improve the services they were providing was just an unnecessary additional burden, on an already overloaded system.

We thought that working top down would firstly help senior managers feel less threatened, because they would have more understanding than the staff they were managing. Moreover, we also thought that if senior managers were seen to be considering continual improvement as a priority for action, others would find it difficult to relegate continual improvement as a marginal activity.

The second element of our project plan was to ensure that the way we used and introduced the EFQM approach, would be through progressively replacing ineffective management approaches, with more effective approaches based on the principles of excellence described by the EFQM Model.

By slowly merging the EFQM process with the day to day management process, the implementation process could be managed within the limited resources we had. In addition, by frequently reflecting on what worked and did not work, the approach could be progressively fine tuned to the needs of the Trust.

The approach would then be spread progressively deeper into the organisation through coaching, self-assessment and reviews. This would be integrated directly into the normal clinical and management processes of the Trust and would build on the tools and techniques already used by many staff across the organisation.

The implementation plan and approaches used would be periodically evaluated by the participants in the process and the approach and project plan modified in the light of that feedback. In this way the approach would reflect real experiences rather than meaningless arbitrary objectives. In addition, by involving the participants in the process of planning and implementation, the approaches used would develop more ownership and commitment to what was being done.

1.7   Training and education on implementation.

Formal training would be provided to meet specific needs on a just-in-time basis in order to increase attendance and transfer new ideas into practice.
While the Trust was developing our concept and approach to the introduction of the EFQM approach to self assessment and review, it is important to recognise that the training in quality management and its tools and techniques were ongoing across the Trust. In November, 1994 the Clinical Nurse Manager for General Medicine suggested that the Trust's training on quality management which at the time was targeted at clinical directors, heads of department, business managers and ward staff, should be given a certificate in recognition of that training. This was introduced on 18th November 1994, for those staff who had taken part in Quality Development Team training and had implemented a quality improvement as a result of that training.

In addition to quality improvement tools and techniques training, we introduced in collaboration with the Management School of the University of

Salford, workshops on the Trust's approach to quality management together with an overview of quality management tools and techniques. These workshops were targeted at the Trust Clinical Management Teams, established when the Trust became formally self-managing in April, 1994. The final workshop was held on 10th February, 1995.

The workshops were delivered by myself as the Trust's Corporate Development Manager and the Director of the Management Development Unit, at the University of Salford.

1.8 Workshop content

The workshops focused on:

- **a review of the principles of the Trust's approach to quality management**
- **an overview of core quality management tools and techniques**
- **an opportunity to identify current issues and problems which the clinical management teams needed to solve**
- **a problem solving process with techniques for analysing systems: i.e. Control Charts, Deployment Flow Charts, Cause and Effect Charts**
- **an agreement as to actions and timescales.**

These workshops led to a flurry of improvement activities across the Trust and where the leadership was good such as in Diabetes and Endocrinology, the pay back was sustained and significant. The improvement activities within the Diabetes services were led by their consultant who played a significant part in developing the Trust's approach to quality management and more importantly in turning that approach into a notable exemplar of excellence in practice.

1.9 An example within the Diabetes Service

The diabetes service in 1994 had a number of serious problems, which included an increase in the rate of complaints from diabetic patients. The diabetes team recognised that any solution could only be effective, if multidisciplinary working across the primary-secondary divide was strengthened.

Their analysis led to the conclusion that they needed to establish 100% shared care between primary and secondary care staff, which could only be achieved if they could create a local diabetes register accessible to those staff. This was duly established and now all patients receive an annual clinical review by a doctor and a nurse in either the hospital or community, depending on their 'type' of diabetes. Any problems occurring between the reviews were referred to a specialist nurse for assessment.

The impact of these developments have been dramatic. The percentage of patients screened within the twelve month period for 1998 was 73% compared to 55% in 1993. The result was a reduction in patients with total cholesterol of <5.5 mmols/l from 32% in 1993 to 74% in 1998 and an increase in patients total LDL cholesterol of < 3.5 mmols/l from 15% in 1993 to 54% in 1998. Of most significance was a reduction in number of diabetes related below-knee amputations from 9 in 1993 to 4 in 1998 and a reduction in diabetes related amputations of toes from 15 in 1993 to 8 in 1998. Furthermore, the national rate for blindness due to diabetes is between 1-4% while Salford, which is a socially and economically deprived area, has only 0.04%.

Personally speaking, the diabetes team exemplified excellence in health care and their practice also mirrored the key elements of the EFQM Model. There was clear and strong leadership which used a coaching and facilitative style. Policy and strategy was developed by the team and there was a clear system of training to enable staff to deliver their services effectively. Processes were reviewed and improved. The results were orientated towards patients' needs, and high standards were expected by staff. The results included satisfaction and clinical outcomes and access to the service and all within a balanced budget. This commitment and continuous improvement is still a strong feature within the diabetes services, demonstrating clearly the impact that leadership on people, policy and strategy and partnerships & resources could have on processes, which impacts on results and performance of value to people and customers alike. In sum, it is a clear indication of how the EFQM Excellence Model could provide a framework for 'sustainable continuous improvement'.

Clearly, leadership together with using the right tools and techniques was the secret of success. The problem for the Trust was how to ensure all clinical and managerial leaders operated at this level.

1.10 Using the EFQM approach to strengthen leadership and deliver the results.

Having completed this training, it was clear that the EFQM Model provided an opportunity to bring together all the quality initiatives that were already in use, as well as being capable of integrating future initiatives. This latter point was critically important for at that time, the Trust was being bombarded with initiative after initiative from the NHS Executive and the Department of Health. Not surprisingly, there was an overwhelming reluctance to progress from one short term initiative to another. We recognised that the EFQM Model could provide an overarching framework for any and every initiative that could be imposed upon us. It also meant that we could handle any new initiative, maintaining a single conceptual framework that supported a consistent long term strategy, with the key aim of creating a culture of quality and excellence.

A culture of excellence can be seen as one in which all staff are involved and committed to achieving long term excellence. Such excellence should be applicable to clinical, academic and service provision for all health care stakeholders, through evidence based decision making which would lead to economic, efficient, effective, equitable and ethical outcomes, within an overarching coaching and facilitative leadership style. The European Foundation for Quality Management (EFQM) Model provided a methodology for assessing our progress towards this culture of excellence over time, something which we had lacked previously.

1.11   Initial steps.

The Trust first used the Model to gain a general overview of the organisation using a series of semi-structured interviews with key staff. The interviews focused on issues relating to how the organisation was performing, compared to the characteristics identified in the Model. Other sources of performance information were also examined against EFQM criteria.

This initial picture of the organisation was then compiled into a list of organisational strengths and areas for improvement, and circulated to members of the Management Board.

The Board met to discuss this initial organisational self-assessment and agreed the Trust's key strengths and areas for improvement. There was an intention to calculate a baseline score for the organisation, in order to help emphasise the key areas of weakness in the organisation, which would then be targeted for improvement by the Board. These target areas for improvement would be agreed with a responsible officer from the Board. Progress would then be reviewed monthly. These areas for improvement were then to be scored individually in order to measure the effectiveness of the agreed action plan. A review schedule was to be agreed and after 12 months the cycle would be repeated.

In 1994, the Trust made explicit the benefits expected from using the EFQM Model as follows:

- to gain a thorough understanding of the strengths and areas for improvement of the organisation as a whole and in its parts
- to provide an action plan prioritised according to identified needs
- to provide a benchmark against world class organisation
- to gain consensus as to what had been achieved and what still needed to be done
- to provide an objective review of progress
- to enable all staff to contribute to the assessment and organisational review process
- to integrate quality improvement into to every aspect of organisational performance.

A semi-structured questionnaire was developed in December 1994 and interviews with the Trust's Management Board members and a cross section of clinicians, was completed by the end of January 1995.

The assessment provided a detailed 28 page report on key strengths and areas for improvement and was the first time that such a detailed picture of the Trust's strengths and areas for improvement was available for strategic management purposes. In many ways however, the detail and comprehensiveness was more of a problem than a help, as it raised so many problem areas, that it was difficult to decide which were the priority for improvement action.

The overall assessment found that there was some evidence that the Trust's approach to management was based on continual improvement methodologies. Especially strong, was the structured devolution of decision making and significant involvement of clinicians in the management process. There was also a systematic approach to the development of clinical and non-clinical quality performance, through the Trust's quality management system. However, integration with and deployment of continual improvement methods within the key processes of the organisation were in an early stage of development. Most management activity was still reactive to problems rather than proactive and being based on early detection and prevention systems.

The Trust's results showed some improvement trends in key Patient Charter standards and the financial results were showing the required overall income expenditure balance. However, the Trust did not have an agreed set of clinical performance results as a target and there were no financial systems for agreeing the best investment decisions, in order to improve the overall Trust's performance.

The findings were presented to the Management Board on 27th February 1995. The short presentation was followed by questions about the Model and the assessment's findings. The key feature which the Management Board found attractive was how the Model had enabled the organisation to focus on key results, in particular clinical results. Prior to that, Management Board meetings had rarely if ever, discussed clinical results and how they could be improved. Clinical performance was hidden from top management, who generally assumed that clinical staff would know what their key clinical results were.

At the February 1995 meeting, the Management Board formally confirmed the use of the Excellence Model, as the Trust's framework for all clinical and non-clinical management throughout the Trust. The task now was to roll out the use of self-assessment using the EFQM Excellence Model, to all Directorates and the large departments, such as the rehabilitation services etc. Even at this stage, the plan was to progressively move from Directorates to ward level, but only after the Directorate management teams felt confident and competent in using the Model to frame their management practice. There was concern to ensure that senior staff felt comfortable with the approach, before involvement of more junior staff in order not to undermine the authority of the senior staff.

1.12 Lessons fom America; March 1995.

In March, the Executive Medical Director and the Quality Manager were asked by the local Health Authority to visit America's leading hospitals to identify performance indicators in use, and how they managed their organisations to deliver improved clinical care. Leading hospitals were chosen either because of their reputation such as the Mayo Clinic, or because they had been winners of state quality awards based on the criteria of the Malcolm Baldrige National Quality Award, such as Florida Medical Centre.

The visit provided much food for thought and a series of key conclusions in relation to the future EFQM implementation were drawn as follows:

quality management needed to be part of the normal management arrangements of the organisation and not an add-on, operating in parallel to the rest of the management system;

clinicians needed to lead improvement processes if they were to realise the potential clinical and cost improvement opportunities;

improvement activity needed to be encouraged and rewarded if best practice was to be developed and shared with others;

there needed to be a common framework through which performance could be made visible and through which the mission and strategic objectives could be communicated and reviewed.

A key warning on implementation also came through and that was; *'only a few people will quickly recognise the value of the approach'*. Most will struggle with the changes and skill development required and a few will attempt to block progress. The secret of successful rapid implementation was summarised by the President and Chief Executive of Florida Medical Centre, when he advised that we:

'Carry the wounded and shoot the stragglers'.

Though amused by the advice, Salford was happy to carry its wounded but had no stomach for shooting stragglers. We worked with the interested, supported those who found the process difficult and ignored the stragglers, some of whom still work within the organisation.

As a direct result of the American visit, the Management and Trust Boards adopted the following recommendations:

- *that the Management Board should make quality development its prime concern and thus would take on the role and responsibility which the initial steering group for quality, the HCQM team had taken. This was thought to signal to the Trust, that EFQM would be at the heart of the management process and not another peripheral short term quality initiative.*

- *the Trust's quality improvement team's activities would remain a central part of the Trust's approach to process improvement and would be strengthened by a Quality Award system, in which staff at all levels would be encouraged and gain recognition for improvements to the services which they participated in. The Trust also adopted the 'storyboard format' for sharing these improvements with others.*

- *that a proforma be developed for use in self-assessments which would eventually contain all the key performance data arranged into the EFQM criteria. This should reflect the requirements of clinicians and managers at all levels within the Trust and should be possible to aggregate in such a way that it would provide an over-all Trust self-assessment. This in turn would be used for strategy development and business planning.*

1.13 A programme of initial training and awareness for Directorate and Departmental Teams (April-July, 1995)

Experience of the use of the full model with the Management Board led to a number of conclusions which were to affect the next stage in the implementation of the EFQM process. The first was that a full self-assessment consisting of many pages of strengths and areas for improvement would appear overwhelming and would be off putting to both clinicians and managers, who may interpret this as a paper exercise. The second key conclusion was that by starting with Leadership, the results focus of the Model would become lost, within the long lists of approaches that were not clearly linked to any result.

In addition, it was clear that to use the EFQM Model effectively would require significant amounts of training. But it was also clear that it would be difficult to provide such training which necessitated taking teams out of the work situation for days at a time. This would consequently have disrupted the ability of the Trust to deliver its services. Furthermore classroom based training was not seen as effective in developing transferable skills for the work situation. At the core of our approach was a desire and intention of wanting EFQM to be used as a management skill and not a theoretical concept.

The training strategy that was decided upon was to be one in which there would be a series of short training sessions, followed by coaching and facilitation in the field, followed by reflections on learning and further training on a just-in-time basis.

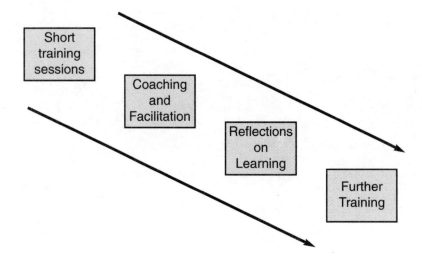

However, such an approach was thought to be incapable of introducing the full complexity of the Model at one time. Neither was it considered necessary to use all the sub-criterion parts of the Model to effectively use it to improve clinical and managerial performance, because using the basic concepts of the model was sufficiently powerful on their own. The full Model would be progressively introduced as clinicians and managers needed to be challenged further in their own skill development and in improving managerial practice within their field of work. Our thinking here was based on the premise that learning is more likely to take place when the learner sees a clear need.

1.14 The training programme

Two hours was assigned to the introductory roll out workshops with the following structure:

Hour 1	Basic concepts of EFQM Model
Hour 2	Self assessment using proforma in Fig 1

 The first hour introduced the basic concepts of the EFQM Model and the second started the process of self-assessment, using the simplified model proforma (Fig. 1). Four sessions were held in which between 10 and 15 senior clinical and managerial staff attended each session. Most who attended were interested in learning more about improving managerial practice, but there were also a proportion of sceptics.

Fig. 1 Performance Management & Review System Self-Assessment Form

This performance management system provides the basis for involving all staff in assessing their own performance, agreeing improvement plans, implementing change and reviewing the effects of those changes. It forms the basis of the formal annual review which ensures appropriate targeting of effort onto key Trust issues, whilst at the same time ensuring that the Trust's priorities match local priorities and requirements.

ASSESSMENT CRITERIA: For each of the assessment criteria, you should identify both your directorates/departments strengths and areas for improvement:

REFERENCE DOCUMENT: Specify the source of data/information on performance for each of the strengths and areas for improvement identified.

SCORING CRITERIA: Using the source document, give a score for each strength/area for improvement specified:

0 - No reference document or anecdotal evidence of performance
1 - Measurable evidence of performance but shows deteriorating trend over the past two years
2 - Measurable evidence of performance but shows deteriorating trend over past year
3 - Measurable evidence of performance and shows steady state over past year
4 - Measurable evidence of performance and shows improving trend over past year
5 - Measurable evidence of performance and shows improving trend for last two years or more.

PRIORITISATION: Class each of the strengths/areas for improvement specified as:

A - Critical to the success of the service and must demonstrate improvement within the next 12 months.

B - Critical to the success of the service and must demonstrate improvement within the next 3 years.

C - Critical to the success of the service but no urgency to demonstrate improvements

D - Not critical to the success of the service but would like to improve if resources became available.

E - Should do when opportunity arises.

KEY PERFORMANCE RESULTS

Q1: Consider the core purpose of your directorate/department in terms of :
(a) How effective it is.
(b) How satisfied those to whom you provide the service are.
(c) How well your service contributes to better personal, community and environmental health.

KEY PROCESSES

Q2 Name the key processes you manage and specify the procedures/protocols which ensure that they are reviewed and continuously improved.

Q3 Specify the key processes which have been improved during the last 12 months.

Q4 Specify the improvement that have been introduced to reduce risks to staff, patients and visitors.

KEY RESOURCES

Q5 Specify the procedures/protocols which are used to ensure optimum use of financial, materials, buildings, equipment and suppliers used by your directorate/department.

Q6 Specify the improvements to the quality of information used for monitoring and decision making which have been made during the last 12 months.

Q7 Specify what new technologies/methods of working which have been introduced to improve performance and market position.

KEY HUMAN RESOURCE ISSUES

Q8 Specify the procedures/protocols which you use to involve staff in agreeing targets, reviewing performance and implementing continuous improvement.

Q9 Specify the extent to which you have implemented policies on recruitment, training, development and career progression.

Q10 Specify the extent to which effective top-down and bottom-up communication is in place.

KEY LEADERSHIP ISSUES

Q11 Specify the ways top management team are personally and visibly involved in leading and promoting quality systems, in line with the Trust's quality objectives.

Q12 Specify the ways the top management team are actively involved in ensuring that patients, purchasers and G.Ps. views are addressed and their reasonable expectations are met.

KEY POLICY & STRATEGY ISSUES

Q13 Specify the key elements of your business plan which will aim to improve your service and help achieve the Trust's objectives during the next 12 months.

Q14 Specify how you will monitor and review progress in the achievement of your objectives and business plan during the next 12 months.

ASSESSMENT CRITERIA	REFERENCE DOCUMENT	SCORE	IMPROVEMENT PRIORITY
1 **KEY PERFORMANCE RESULTS** (Non-financial): Specify the key indicators you need to determine the effectiveness of the service you provide - include how you would be assessed in terms of the Trust's key objectives, your profession's standards/research, purchaser requirements and the satisfaction levels of patients and other users of your service: **Strengths:** **Areas for Improvement:**			

1.15   Areas for improvement:

These short training sessions revealed that only a few clinicians and managers were clear about what their key results should be. However, surgeons were much clearer about the type of indicators which they would like to have measured, than were most other clinical groups. They were more able to specify activities which they carried out. But they often considered success more as completion of task that they had been given to do, rather than how well these tasks had impacted on key results required by the Trust's mission or of requirements of customers and other stakeholders.

The process made visible, key weaknesses in many manager's and clinician's approaches to management. The strong message given was that this should not be seen as a personal criticism, but as an opportunity to learn more effective ways of managing. It was thought that if self-assessment was to be effective, it needed to be done in a safe environment in which people would openly recognise the areas in which they needed to improve.

 Following these sessions, ongoing coaching and facilitation was provided to those who wanted it. While most took advantage of this offer, there were others who did not. Most clinicians and managers reacted to the learning opportunity and strengthened their own management approaches. The best self-assessments took on the form of action learning groups led by the senior clinician or manager. Overall improvement activities, which had stalled prior to the introduction of the quality awards as part of the EFQM process, increased. However, others made little effort to use the process to strengthen their own management practices. Instead they continued to rely on their traditional 'fire fighting' approaches, with no effect on improving service performance.

A review of the self-assessments revealed how little understanding there was of the mission of the organisation and how their individual roles and responsibilities contributed to that mission. It also demonstrated that information systems in existence then, were poorly orientated to the needs of clinicians and managers. Rather these information systems seemed to be designed to provide information to external monitoring bodies, focusing on their specific agendas. The limited information resources of the Trust were thus put under greater pressure by an increasing need for information, to improve the clinical and managerial processes of the Trust, whilst at the same time facing up to increase demand for information, external to the Trust.

The self-assessments however started to provide for the first time, a set of key performance indicators which both clinicians and managers feel were meaningful and helpful in terms of managing their services, in order to meet their patients' needs. A set of indicators was progressively developed and an extract from the results section of these is given in Fig 2.

Fig 2

EFQM9b	Organisational Results - non financial		
	Corporate Clinical Indicators		
OR(b)C1	Percentage of Clinical Directorates which can demonstrate improvement trends in at least one key	Clinical Performance Managers	Bi-annually
OR(b)C1 (NCEI)	28 day emergency re-admission rates	Management Information	Quarterly
OR(b)C2 (NCEI)	In-hospital adverse drug related events	Clinical Audit	Bi-annually
	Surgical Specialities Group **Clinical Indicators**		
OR(b)S1	Percentage of Caesarean Section Deliveries (Obstetrics)	Management Information	Quarterly
OR(b)S2a	Five year survival rates for cancers of ovary (Gynaecology)	Clinical Audit	Bi-annually
OR(b)S2b	Five year survival rates for cancers of ovary (Gynaecology)	Clinical Audit	Bi-annually
OR(b)S2c (NCEI)	Five year survival rates for cancers of cervix (Gynaecology)	Clinical Audit	Bi-annually
OR(b)S3	Ratio of Forceps to Ventose (Obstetrics)	Management Information	Quarterly
OR(b)S4	Occurrence of Maternal Deaths (Obstetrics)	Management Information	Annually
OR(b)S5 (NCEI)	Stillbirth rate per 1000 births (Obstetrics)	Management Information	Quarterly
OR(b)S6 (NCEI)	Comparison of <40 to 40 > 40 patients with (D&C) as primary procedure (Gynaecology)	Management Information	Quarterly
OR(b)S7	Number of Hysterectomies (Gynaecology)	Management Information	Annually
OR(b)S8	Re-admission following Termination of Pregnancy (Gynaecology)	Management Information	Annually
OR(b)S10	X-ray reporting response times (Radiology)	Clinical Audit	Monthly
OR(b)S11	Percentage use of I/V sedation in Oral Surgery (Oral Surgery)	Clinical Audit	Quarterly
OR(b)S12	Oesophago-gastrectromy mortality rates (General Surgery and Surgical Gastroenterology) (within stay)	Management Information	Bi-annually
OR(b)S13	Leak rates following excision of colon (General Surgery and Surgical Gastroenterology)	Clinical Audit	Bi-annually

In May 1995, guidance on how the self-assessments would form the basis of the performance management of the Trust was issued. The heart of this process would be a corporate self-assessment carried out annually by the Management Board. During the year each directorate/business unit using the Model would assess its own strengths and areas for improvement. These local self assessments would then form the basis of an annual performance review, in which the local management team would agree their self assessment and key areas for improvement, with their senior manager/clinical director as shown in Fig 3.

Fig 3 SELF ASSESSMENT REVIEWER RESPONSIBILITY

QUARTER	SELF ASSESSMENT TEAM	REVIEWER
JUL-AUG	BUSINESS UNIT/WARD/DEPARTMENT	CLINICAL DIRECTOR/ MANAGER
SEP-OCT	CLINICAL DIRECTORATE MANAGEMENT TEAM	MEDICAL DIRECTOR/ GENERAL MANAGER
NOV-DEC	MEDICAL DIRECTOR/EXECUTIVE DIRECTOR /GENERAL MANAGER	CHIEF EXECUTIVE
DEC-JAN	MANAGEMENT BOARD	TRUST BOARD

These local self-assessment would provide part of the data for the corporate self assessment process and therefore needed to be an honest appraisal of what local strengths and weaknesses were. Weaknesses were to be considered as opportunities for improvement and no blame or judgements about fault was to be made at any stage in the review process. This review system was also about exploring together, ways of continually improving the service; it was not about finding faults with those who worked in that service.

Using the agreed self assessment profile of the organisation, the Management and Trust Board would go on to agree the strategic and business plans for the Trust. Key performance targets would be identified by the Trust and incorporated into the local self assessment profile and business plans.

For each key target area, performance indicators were to be defined and monitoring systems established. It was thought that there needed to be three levels of performance information:

Level 1   Specific/individual performance data

Level 2   Speciality/Directorate/Departmental aggregated data

Level 3   Corporate aggregated data

Level 1 data was required for individual monitoring and problem solving. Level 2 data for operational management and control and level 3, for corporate monitoring and control.

Level 3 performance indicators would be reported in the Corporate Performance Report to the Executive Group during the 2nd Monday of each month, and the Management Board on the 3rd Monday of each month.

Data related to the Corporate Performance report would be collected via Management Information, who would also monitor Level 2 and Level 1 indicators which had been used in the data aggregation process. Areas of concern determined as performance falling outside control/action limits, or showing a strong tendency towards them, would be highlighted. When this occurred, additional information in the form of level 1 or 2 run charts (ie Pareto), would be included in the Corporate Performance Report, so that responsibility for ensuring corrective action to be taken could be allocated. The Executive Group/Management Board would produce an action plan (Fig. 4) to address areas of concern raised in these Corporate Performance Report.

Circulation of the Corporate Performance Report together with appropriate Level 1 and 2 information, would be via Directorate Performance Managers, who would receive the information on the last Monday of the month following the month being monitored. Local review of performance together with local action plans, would be agreed with performance managers at their local monthly performance review meetings.

Fig 4

ACTION PLAN:

REQUIRED OUTCOME	REPORT FORMAT	ACTION & RESPONSIBILITY	DATE GIVEN	SCHEDULE CHECK	DATE DUE	COMMENTS

All Quality Development Teams (QDT'S) were to be led by the process owner and given clear deadlines and authority to improve the system. Core membership of the team had to reflect the key elements of the process. Members were co-opted as necessary, to fully analyse and identify the 'best' solutions. All QDT's were expected to give a final report no later than 120 days after the start of the project, with an interim report at the halfway stage.

All improvement had also to be submitted for consideration for the Trust Board's Quarterly Award, for the best quality improvement to the service. These submissions were to be short-listed by the Trust's Executive Management using the following criteria:

- Quality/financial improvements achieved
- Importance to the Trust
- News value
- Sustainability
- Transferability.

The final winner was to be selected and presented with the award by the Chief Executive and Trust Chairman, following an exhibition of the short-listed entries. All submissions for the award had to be through the Corporate Development Manager.

This performance management system was a process for involving all staff in assessing their own performance, agreeing improvement plans, implementing changes, reviewing the effects of those changes and sharing success and learning with colleagues across the Trust. In addition, the approach allowed for measures of progress to be made and good practice highlighted for external publicity purposes. At the same time, the formal review process used a coaching/facilitating management style, to ensure that there was appropriate targeting of effort onto key issues while at the same time not stifling local aspirations. Such an approach to performance management, was designed to unlock the highest levels of self motivation and creativity amongst all the staff employed by the Trust, for the benefit of patients and staff alike.

1.16 Facilitator Training July 1995

In order to provide local support for the implementation of the Trust's quality management approach, a series of intensive training programs were provided for a selected group of interested staff, within each of the key management groupings of the Trust. Their role was:

- *to promote the Trust's quality management philosophy and methodology of management in order to ensure a systematic and continual search for:*

-**Quality development**
-**Optimisation of resource utilisation**
-**Risk reduction**

- *to provide independent facilitation and support to quality development teams (QDT's), working in parts of the organisation in which the facilitator had no line management responsibilities.*

- *to help QDT's by:*

-**providing training in quality management tools and techniques**
-**supporting team structured problem solving and project management**
-**cultivating teamwork**
-**coaching the team leader**

- *to develop further skills in quality management and facilitation through membership of an action learning set of other facilitators, meeting for 2 hours per fortnight.*

1.17   Person specification for Facilitators.

In order to attract, staff of the right calibre, a list of specifications was drawn up as follows:-

- knowledge of the Trust's quality management philosophy and methodology
- experience of leading teams and introducing quality improvements.*
- well respected by both senior and junior staff.*
- coaching and facilitating style of leadership.*
- excellent listening and communicating skills.*
- excellent time management skills.*
- good understanding of statistics and data analysis.
- self confident and highly motivated.*
- thorough understanding of the organisation's structures and functions.
- able to commit at least 3 hours per week to this role, including 2 hours per fortnight facilitator development, as part of an action learning set.*

Those marked with '*' were the minimum requirements prior to selection for training. However, it was unlikely that any candidate would have all the attributes required, but it was anticipated that the full range of attributes would be developed through action learning, facilitated by the Corporate Development Manager.

1.18   Facilitator development programme

The introductory program lasted two days with twelve people attending. The program included:

role of the facilitator in health care quality management
overview of facilitation
attributes of a facilitator
team roles and dynamics
leadership and facilitation (Skill Building)
problem solving tools and techniques.

The invitation to apply went out under the Chief Executive's name and Heads of Departments had to agree to release their nominated staff, for a minimum of three hours per week to this role. There was a positive response and we had fifteen nominations.

1.19   Quality awards for innovations and improvements April, 1995

In April 1995, the Management Board approved the establishment of the Trust Quality Awards in order to give recognition and encouragement to those who were motivated to improve their services and as an encouragement to others, to become interested in continuous improvement.

It was clear that the work done to introduce TQM into the Trust had not been able to show any clear evidence of impact. This was thought to be due to the absence of mechanisms, to collect and share the improvement introduced.

1.20   First Chief Executive Reviews (1996)

The initial intention was to hold the reviews of the directorate and departmental self-assessments on an annual basis, in order to confirm the commitment of the Trust's top management team to the self-assessment process and to use the self-assessments as the basis for strategic and business planning. There was a considerable delay before the first Chief Executive Review took place, because the quality manager wanted the self-assessments to be performed to a high standard before the reviews took place. This was a mistake for two reasons. The first was that those who had progressed the self-assessments did not get early feedback on how well they were doing. The second was that a number of managers delayed doing theirs until they were convinced that this was seen as important by the Chief Executive, which was to be signalled by the review itself.

The first review was fairly informal and much more of a joint learning and coaching exercise than a review. The purpose of the first review was to find an effective and acceptable approach for all parties. The adoption of a joint learning style to the review was effective in making the review seen as a helpful process rather than a judgmental process. The Chief Executive spent about half a day on each review with each team and together a deeper understanding of the organisation, the Excellence Model and how to make the most effective use of the approach developed. The review process also reinforced the commitment of the top team to the process and helped to ensure that aspirations of departments identified through their self-assessment, could be better matched to the strategic needs and capabilities of the Trust as a whole.

1.21 EFQM Review Workshop: September, 1996

At the end of the first set of reviews, a workshop was held in order to:

- to identify and share best practice and key learning points in using the EFQM self-assessment method.
- to introduce the core performance indicator set for use across the Trust, as part of the performance management system.
- to agree targets for the integration of the EFQM self-assessment process with the business planning and budget setting cycle.

The program included an introduction to the workshop and its objectives led by the Chief Executive. This was followed by case presentations and reflections on the self-assessment and review process, led by the lead for each of the Trust's major management groupings: Medicine, Surgery, Finance, Information, Human Resources and Facilities. The final session consisted of an open discussion session, led by the Chief Executive. A number of key learning points came out of this workshop. The first was that some people had difficulty in understanding the difference between results and enablers. In addition, a significant number struggled with defining indicators of performance.

Furthermore, only a few departments and directorates were clear about how their activity contributed to the overall mission and strategy of the organisation. In particular, there was a lack of key performance measures for clinical effectiveness and an absence of measures for customer and people satisfaction.

In terms of the process used by the Trust, a number of key lessons emerged. The first reinforced the need for increasing amounts of training, not simply in terms of the use of the EFQM Model, but in basic managerial skills such as clarifying results, determining key processes, communication, change management, action planning and implementation of improvement action through teams.

There was a general appeal for more prescription from the top as to what the key indicators should be. However, there was also the recognition that the lack of prescription did help them to be more able to generate new and more appropriate indicators for their services.

The central importance of the Chief Executive review as a process for motivating, coaching and learning was strongly confirmed and was therefore increased from an annual to six monthly basis, because of the need to keep the EFQM process at the forefront of manager's minds.

The introduction of a simplified version of the Model, initially helped users to focus on the key concepts of good management practice implicit in the Model, in such a way that managers and clinicians did not feel overwhelmed with the apparent complexity of the Model.

1.22   Strengthening the process (1997 - 1998)

Following the first reviews, there was an increasing demand to use the whole model at directorate and departmental level. The full model together with training was provided, together with an increasing number of staff attending the EFQM or BQF Licensed Assessor programme.

The demand by most managers for the use of the full model rather than the simplified model, led us to develop our original proforma further. An example of the new proforma is shown in Fig 5. In addition, more detailed guidance on what was expected in a full self-assessment was given.

In carrying out the assessment the following documents were expected to be used:

- The Trust's Strategic and Business Plans.
- The department's business/service plan.
- Standards of Service (A document summarising all of the Trust's standards).
- Performance reports.
- Service level agreements and contracts.
- Corporate Indicator Set.

It was anticipated that the first complete reviews would take a significant amount of time to complete. This was the original reason for using a shortened form, but the enthusiasm at the time for using the full model meant that this was not considered to be an impediment at this stage. In addition, the use of a proforma would mean that future self-assessments would be done rapidly, because all that would be needed would be updates to the performance data and a few amendments to the areas being addressed. At first, filling in the detail did take a great deal of time, but now the process is very fast because only additions or amendments need to be added in order to bring the self-assessment up to date.

The key messages given were that in assessing the results, teams should first consider their non-financial results. Here they were expected to specify their strengths and areas for improvement, in terms of the key indicators of the effectiveness of their service and note the reference documents that could be used to validate the self-assessment. For clinical services, they were expected to consider the type of clinical outcome or health gain indicators that they would like to use. For non-clinical areas, they needed to specify the quality and delivery performance of the service or products that they provided.

Once clear about their key results in terms of each criteria of the Excellence Model, the teams were asked to consider their key enablers. These were described as the structures and processes which made it possible to deliver their key results.

Starting with the key processes which were central to the achievement of their key results, managers and clinicians were asked to consider how well their service's practices adhered to procedures, protocol and guidelines which had been issued. They also had to consider how their activities compared to the best practices reported in the professional journals, research reports and standards of service which applied to their department. They were also expected to consider how they managed risks within the service provided.

Fig 5

Criteria Part:
(insert criteria spcification)

Area to Address	Performance Indicator	Performance and Deployment Trend Summary	Reference Document	Comment: (Strength/area for improvement/issues to be addressed)	Agreed action following review
(insert area being addressed)	(Insert key process and indicator of its performance)	(Insert summary of performance trend and the extent to which the process is deployed to its potential)			

They also had to assess how they ensured that they had the staff necessary for the achievement of their results and how effectively they used their skills and involved them in decision making. In addition, they were asked to consider how effectively they motivated and trained their staff and how well their processes of two way communication functioned.

In addition, they were challenged as to how well they managed their material, equipment and facilities and how they have tried to achieve the optimum level of efficiency, through being kept up to date with technological and methodological advances.

They were also asked to consider their own leadership team's strengths and areas for improvement. And finally, they had to specify the improvement targets they had set for their service, both the short term (12 months) and long term (2-5 years).

A good self-assessment was to be a balanced picture of the service's strengths and areas for improvement. In addition, the results had to have sufficient scope to include all the indicators by which service performance could be assessed. The enabler section was concerned with the effectiveness of the approach and the extent to which it was deployed in all the appropriate areas of the service.

The importance and value of the Chief Executive review was such that the Trust decided that these reviews should be held at six monthly intervals, rather than annually. These self-assessments were to become the basis of the Trust's new performance management system (Fig 6).

Fig 6

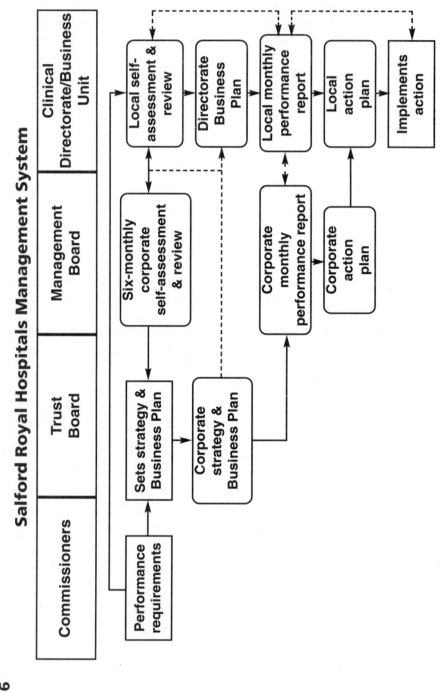

Salford Royal Hospitals Management System

The local self-assessments were to be the source of local business/service plans. These would lead onto departmental/directorate performance management systems, based on the improvement cycle of monthly monitoring of performance through local performance reports. These in turn would lead to improvement actions, the effectiveness of which would be assessed by their impact on performance.

Local self-assessments would be aggregated and compiled into a corporate self-assessment which would form the basis of the corporate business plan. This in turn would be monitored by the Management Board through monthly monitoring reports. Corporate action plans would be issued to specific members of the Management Board, who would then implement these as part of their local performance management system.

On a six monthly basis, each department/directorate would review how well it had progressed towards excellence as conceptualised by the EFQM Model. This would be reviewed by the group General Manager, Medical Director and other chosen members of their review team. These departmental/directorate reviews would then be aggregated to form the basis of a group self-assessment, which would form the basis of the six monthly Chief Executive Reviews.

A number of managers felt that they wanted to develop their own proforma, to reflect their own needs and increase ownership of the process. This was agreed to and a number of variations of the corporate proforma (Fig. 5) were developed. However, most used the corporate proforma.

General Managers and Directors were given the responsibility to determine how the process was to be implemented into their areas of responsibility. Support was provided as needed from the trained facilitators. Each major management grouping had at least one of these.

The numbers of staff trained to the level of EFQM or BQF Licensed assessor also increased. The Licensed Assessor program was felt to increase the depth of understanding of the Model and good management practice and also strengthened commitment to the process of the facilitators.

The most effective users of the Model managed to ensure that their self-assessment became part of their business planning process. They also preferred to use the self-assessment as the business planning submission document, rather than the traditional business plan which they used to submit and which most found of little value. The Contracting and Business Planning

Directorate agreed that they would accept the self-assessment, rather than the traditional business plan for future business planning purposes.

The most effective users also consulted their staff over the content of the self-assessment and used it to coach their staff in understanding the process and the good management practices, that it highlighted. One of the best early users of this was the rehabilitation services, which took time to get all their staff trained and involved them in the self-assessment process. The group has continued to develop the approach and is one of the most prolific quality award participants. A survey of staff carried out within the rehabilitation services found the following:

	before	after
Satisfaction with professional issues	51%	72%
Satisfaction with communication	40%	80%
Accessibility of managers	46%	82%
Usefulness of meetings	21%	52%

1.23 Developments in the Chief Executive Review (1997 -1998)

For most clinicians, managers and directors, the importance of positive feedback and guidance on the next steps given by the Chief Executive was considered to be both a strength and critical aspect of an effective performance management system.

The link between self-assessment and the hospital's business planning, budget setting and performance management system, was to be part of the Chief Executive's Review meeting. During this review, the aspirations of departments/directorates and the strategic needs of the Trust as a whole were matched. In addition, actions were agreed and prioritised and the level of resources requested, confirmed.

During this period, the Chief Executive Review started to take on a distinctive form. A copy of local self-assessment, together with proposed targets for improvements had to be sent to the Chief Executive no later than 14 days prior to the review. In practice this usually arrived only a few days before the review date. This should have included a summary of the self-assessment and the key issues for review/discussion.

At the review meeting, key members of the local management team, including performance manager/facilitator, were expected to attend. In practice most teams included between 5 - 15 people. Those attending considered that it was important for members of the extended management team to meet the Chief Executive and have the opportunity to discuss directly, management issues that they had successfully achieved or had concerns about.

The review tended to take place in three sections and never lasted more than three hours in total:

1.24   Section 1 of the review meeting
The self-assessment team made a brief presentation of identified strengths, areas for improvement and issues it wished to have considered by the review team. This included an outline of how all staff had been involved in the self-assessment process, or how they planned to involve all staff in the future.

1.25   Section 2 of the review meeting
The review team asked questions and made observations about the self-assessment. These questions focused on the extent to which the self-assessment results had:
- *covered all stakeholders*
- *clear improvement targets*
- *measured soft and hard aspects of performance*
- *showed positive and sustained trends*
- *been compared to others e.g. best in class*
- *measured what was important now and in the future*
- *clearly related results to enabler approaches chosen*
- *provided a holistic picture of the service*

Questions on enablers focused on approach and deployment. These included:

was the approach (best practice) chosen:
-dealing with the right priorities?
-effective in achieving the targets set?
-integrated into policy and strategy?
-evidence based?
-prevention based?
-sustainable?
-innovative?
-flexible?
-measurable?

Were the approaches used deployed:
efficiently?
to their full potential?
quickly?
systematically?
understood and accepted by all stakeholders?
measurable?

And finally, did they have a local review process which was carried out regularly, benchmarked with others, improved systematically and used as an opportunity for shared learning?

1.26   Section 3 of the review meeting
Finally, the review team and the self-assessment team agreed improvement targets, cost improvements, investments required and time-scales.

1.27   Corporate (EFQM) Self-assessment Management Board Review Workshop 9th October, 1998
As had become the practice, each Chief Executive Review was followed by a review workshop in order to achieve shared learning and ownership of the process. A significant review workshop was held in October 1998, at which the following key actions (enablers) were agreed:

* *Publish Strategic Direction - April 1999*
* *Strengthen the collective Trust Board ownership of the EFQM process*
* *Improve the coverage of critical issues highlighted through the self-assessment process*
* *Medical Education to be included in future self-assessment and reviews*
* *Involve all clinical directors in a central role in the EFQM self-assessment and review process*
* *Feedback interim review to all clinical directors*
* *Develop mechanisms for personal appraisal of clinical directors*
* *Develop educational programmes to support the cascading of the process of self-assessment and review throughout the organisation, with special emphasis on engaging medical staff in the process*
* *Appropriate Executive Directors to be part of Chief Executives Review team.*

1.28   Key Improvement Priorities for financial year 1999/2000 were to be:

1.28.1   Results (Non-financial)

- *Extend the clinical indicators used by Clinical Directorates*
- *Develop activity and capacity plans for all Clinical Directorates.*

1.28.2   Results (Financial)

- *Develop Value for Money indicators of performance*
- *People Satisfaction*
- *Develop the staff satisfaction survey so as to be able to provide directorate and departmental feedback, on their local performance*
- *Customer Satisfaction*
- *Define customers and their key requirements for satisfaction*
- *Provide a customer satisfaction survey service which provides performance information at directorate and departmental level as well as corporate.*

1.29   Impact on Society

- *Achieve the Health and Safety targets, and Clinical Negligence Scheme standards defined in the Risk Management Strategic Plan.*

1.30   Processes

- *Develop information systems which support clinical activity*
- *Integrate self-assessment with the business planning cycle*
- *Integrate benefits realisation with the self-assessment and review process*
- *Establish Controls Assurance processes.*

1.31   Human Resources

- *Increase competence of Executive Directors, Medical and Clinical Directors, General Managers and key Heads of Department in the EFQM self-assessment and review process.*

1.31.1 Resources

- *Establish benchmarks for key resource utilisation rates*
- *Increase capital for medical equipment*
- *Establish space utilisation and allocation controls.*

1.32 Policy and Strategy

- *Implement the national strategies*
- *Define the Trust's values.*

1.33 Leadership

- *Increase the direct leadership involvement in the self-assessment and review process of Clinical Directors.*

1.34 Deployment Review December 1998

The Trust's policy was to involve all staff in the process of EFQM self-assessment and review. Involvement of staff across the Trust was variable, with extensive involvement in some Directorates/Departments whilst others, particularly clinical staff, had not been fully engaged in the process.

With the EFQM Self-assessment and Review process being at the heart of the Trust's approach to General Management, Business Planning, Risk Management and Clinical Governance, it was now vital that all senior staff were appropriately skilled in the use of Trust EFQM performance management and review system.

Key targets were set for full deployment within the next 36 months and in particular:

100% of departments/directorate to be fully involved in the EFQM self-assessment and review process.

80% of clinical staff to use the Model as part of Clinical Governance.

70% of staff in each directorate to be directly involved in the self-assessment and review process.

80% of users will report that they find the EFQM Model helpful.

This would be achieved by:

All new staff being given a specific introduction to the way the EFQM Model is used within the Trust and an outline of their role within that process.

Staff training programmes provided by the Trust would explicitly show how it supports and links to the Trust's EFQM performance improvement framework.

Personal development plans being structured around the framework of the EFQM Model.

Job descriptions being structured around the framework of the EFQM Model.

All staff receiving a booklet giving guidance on how they can use the EFQM Model to improve their services.

All Trust and Management Board members attending the two day awareness and implementation course.

Performance Managers achieving licensed assessor status.

Clinical Directors and General Managers attending a two day course on 'Using the EFQM Model to Manage within the Trust'. The clinical director's course would focus on the use of the Model within the process of Clinical Governance.

Top team networking with leading edge organisations in the use of the Model, in order to identify best practice for use within the Trust and to position the Trust as the leading health care user of the EFQM Model.

Partnership working in the use of the Model with Health Authorities and PCG's would be increased.

1.35 Impact of the introduction of the new 1999 EFQM Model

The introduction of the new 1999 Model by EFQM, led to the further development of the Trust's self-assessment proforma and confirmed the Trust's approach to using the Model as a performance management, rather than simply a review system. Especially welcomed was the confirmation that the Model should be used through a process which starts with clarifying the results required and leading to a circle of improvement, by the identification of approaches, effectively deployed with regular self-assessment and review, which EFQM called RADAR logic (Fig. 7).

Fig 7   Radar Logic

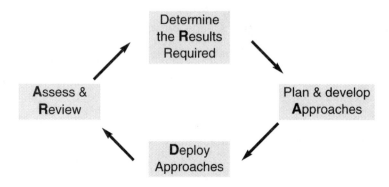

This **RADAR** logic was to be the key to the Trust's management process and was interpreted to apply to the Trust as follows:

Results: Determining and defining the key results the organisation wishes to achieve as part of its policy and strategy making process. For the Trust, these results had to cover how well it was delivering its Mission to achieve clinical, academic and service excellence, financial security and positive perceptions of the Trust by its stakeholders (patients, staff, referring clinicians, commissioners etc.)

Approaches: Planning and developing an integrated set of approaches which were able to deliver these results, both now and in the future.

Deployment: Deploying the approaches selected to their full potential.

Assessment and Review: Achieving organisational learning through assessing and reviewing, the approaches used and their effectiveness in achieving the desired results. Based on this review, prioritising and planning improvement activities needed to achieve continuous improvement.

1.36   Strengthening the focus of the Trust's Management Structure

The management arrangements were developed so as to reflect the key processes of the Trust, based on the EFQM Excellence Model 1999. These arrangements were to provide the structures, through which the roles and responsibilities for key leadership functions could be more effectively discharged.

Fig. 8 outlines the key management processes of the Trust. These processes had a defined set of primary customers. They were further designed to provide an increasingly improving service, through which the Trust Board could discharge its responsibility for Corporate Governance, through the direction and co-ordination of the Management Board.

The Key Customer Facing Processes were those concerned with delivering the mission of the Trust to its external customers, patients, referring clinicians, commissioners of health care and public bodies. These processes were grouped under a defined group management structure. Within each of these, were directorates and departments aligned around a common customer base, such as a clinical speciality including:

Medical Services
Surgical Services
Diagnostic and Therapeutic Services
Research and Development.
Undergraduate/postgraduate and professional clinical education.

It was the responsibility of clinical and managerial leads in each of these areas to continually improve, at an operational level, the requirements of all nine criteria/elements of the EFQM Model.

The Key Support Processes were those which provided support to the Customer Facing Processes in the delivery of the Trust Mission. The primary customers of these processes are the clinical and managerial leads of Key Customer Facing Processes and included:

Human Resources which provide support in achieving excellence in people management defined within the EFQM Model under:

Criterion Three - **People**
Criterion Seven - **People Results**

Finance, Information and Computing that provides support in achieving excellence in non-human resource management, defined within the EFQM Model under:

Criterion Four - **Partnerships and Resources**
Criterion Nine - **Key Performance Results (Financial)**

Contracting and Business Development which provides support in achieving excellence in policy and strategy defined within the EFQM Model under:

Criterion Two - **Policy and Strategy**
Criterion Eight - **Society Results.**

Fig 8

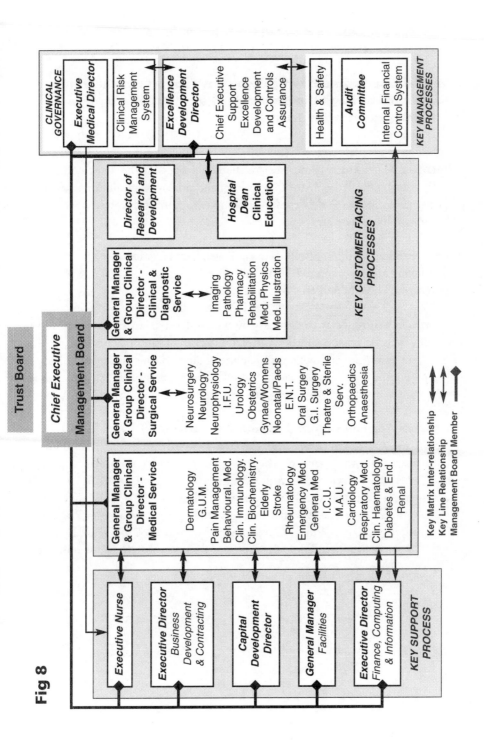

Trust Board

Chief Executive

Management Board

CLINICAL GOVERNANCE

Executive Medical Director

Clinical Risk Management System

Excellence Development Director

Chief Executive Support Excellence Development and Controls Assurance

Health & Safety

Audit Committee

Internal Financial Control System

KEY MANAGEMENT PROCESSES

Director of Research and Development

Hospital Dean Clinical Education

General Manager & Group Clinical Director - Clinical & Diagnostic Service

Imaging
Pathology
Pharmacy
Rehabilitation
Med. Physics
Med. Illustration

General Manager & Group Clinical Director - Surgical Service

Neurosurgery
Neurology
Neurophysiology
I.F.U.
Urology
Obstetrics
Gynae/Womens
Neonatal/Paeds
E.N.T.
Oral Surgery
G.I. Surgery
Theatre & Sterile Serv.
Orthopaedics
Anaesthesia

General Manager & Group Clinical Director - Medical Service

Dermatology
G.U.M.
Pain Management
Behavioural. Med.
Clin. Immunology.
Clin. Biochemistry.
Elderly
Stroke
Rheumatology
Emergency Med.
General Med
I.C.U.
M.A.U.
Cardiology
Respiratory Med.
Clin. Haematology
Diabetes & End.
Renal

KEY CUSTOMER FACING PROCESSES

Executive Nurse

Executive Director Business Development & Contracting

Capital Development Director

General Manager Facilities

Executive Director Finance, Computing & Information

KEY SUPPORT PROCESS

Key Matrix Inter-relationship
Key Line Relationship
Management Board Member

Facilities which provide support in achieving excellence through the provision of supporting facilities.

Capital Development which provides support in achieving excellence through the provision of an appropriate physical infrastructure for the Trust.

The Key Management Processes are the key process of the Trust concerned with assuring the Trust Board that its legal and other obligation for Corporate Governance, are being delivered by those to whom it has devolved operational responsibility. These are:

- Compliance with applicable laws and associated regulations
- Having adequate internal financial controls
- Having efficient and effective operations.

Controls Assurance is the process by which Trust Boards can reassure the public, that the Trust operates an effective system of internal control covering three key risk: clinical, organisational and financial. This is closely linked to the requirement to have efficient and effective operations which are assured through the Trust Performance Management and Review System.

Controls Assurance Clinical - Clinical Governance: This is the process by which the Chief Executive and the Trust Board is assured that there is continuous improvement of the quality of services provided and that standards are safeguarded by the creation of an environment in which excellence in clinical care will flourish. Though the quality of clinical outcomes is the responsibility of individual professional staff, it is the responsibility of the Clinical Governance Committee of the Trust Board to provide an independent controls assurance function for clinical probity and clinical outcomes.

Assurance Financial is the process by which the Chief Executive and the Trust Board are assured that the there is adequate control of the financial resources of the Trust. The Trust's Standing Financial Instructions and other financial policies govern the use by budget holders of the Trust financial resources. Compliance is independently assured through audits, carried out by Internal Audit which reports to the Internal Audit Committee of the Trust Board.

Controls Assurance Organisational is the process by which the Chief Executive and the Trust Board are assured that there is adequate control and co-ordination of the management of all risks facing the Trust. The process is fully described in the Trust's Risk Management System and consists of mechanisms to identify risks, assess and prioritise the relative risk against the Trust's full risk portfolio. It also identifies the appropriate level at which risk management action should be taken and assure the Trust Board, that appropriate decisions in the management of the risks have been taken.

Performance Management and Review is the process by which all staff within the organisation assess their performance against the EFQM framework of organisational excellence. These self-assessments are reviewed by the next in line management team and improvement priorities agreed. Self-assessments and reviews take place through a series of more aggregated levels, moving from individual departments, up to a corporate level assessment which forms the basis of the Trust's business plan. In turn, this is the driver of the performance monitoring and action planning mechanisms.

Within this structure, key managers roles and responsibilities are defined as follows:

Chief Executive: Overall responsibility for strategic and operational management of the Trust and the achievement of its legal and other obligations. The Chief Executive leads the EFQM self-assessment and review process with support form the Executive Directors of the Trust Board and the Excellence Development Director.

Executive Directors: Members of the Trust Board, with joint responsibility for Corporate Governance of the Trust. In addition, they may have responsibility for the management of a particular function or department of the Trust. In this functional role, they are responsible for the achievement of the objectives and the general management of that function, resources and processes.

General Managers: Functional managers responsible for the achievement of the Trust's strategic objectives, through day to day operational management of the resources and processes of a defined grouping of departments/directorates.
Directors: Responsible for the efficient and effective operation of processes which cross defined functional boundaries by providing direction, co-ordination and facilitation to the functional groupings which the process crosses.

Managers: Functional managers responsible for the achievement of the Trust's strategic objectives through day to day operational management of the resources and processes of a defined functional group.

1.37 New proforma 1999

The new Model and review feedback led to the further development of the Trust self-assessment proforma. All directorates are now required to use the new standard format, in order to make aggregation possible and to ensure that all the aspects of good management are covered in the local self-assessment process.

The new proforma attempted to bring together into one place all the information needed to understand what good management required, and provided information on how well the service was performing. It also contained a history of previous performance and action agreed, together with a mechanism to check the extent that those actions had been implemented and had been effective.

Fig. 9 shows part of the results section of the new proforma and an example of a related enabler section. This is based on a real example, though the exact figures have been changed for confidentiality purposes.

Fig 9: Salford Royals Hospitals NHS Trust - Health care Excellence Self-assessment and Review Framework   Key to Framework Codes

Key Performance Results - Key Performance Outcomes (EFQM 9a)
(Key outcomes required by the organisation)

	Results	Trends	Target	Benchmark	Link to Enabler	Comments/Action	Who/When
1	30 day Hospital Mortality rate for Myocardial Infarction	1997 16.0% 1998 14.4%	14.0%	Not available	5d1	*Progress beyond this will require arrangements for thrombolytics to be given in the A&E department.*	CEO/June 2000
2	Budget Variance	1996 =+0.5% 1997 =+0.8% 1998 =-0.1%	0	Not available	4b1, 4b2, & 4b3		
3							

Result number 9a1 Shading indicates CEO key result

Key enabler numbers which are thought to be responsible for this result

Italics indicates this has been added between reviews and is for discussion and agreement at the next review

Bold indicates that this has been added as a requirement following the last review

Additional Results Required and Completion Target Date:

Processes - Products and services are produced, delivered and supported (EFQM 5d)

	Approach	Deployment % Implemented	Measured effectiveness	Improvements Made	Links to Results	Comments/Action	Who/When
1	Thrombolytic therapy within 30 minutes	100% in Heart Care Unit	Percentage of appropriate patients receiving thrombolytics within 30 minutes	1997 = 20% 1998 = 62%	9a1	**Gain agreement to start thrombolytic therapy in the A&E Department**	CEO/June 2000

Additional Approaches/Improvements Required and Completion Target Date:

The following are examples of key indicators of performance used within the self-assessment process within the new proforma:

9a   *Key performance outcomes: (The achievements of the organisation in terms of its planned outcomes)*

e.g.   *30 day peri-operative mortality rates*
Total FCE's
Income expenditure ratio
Number of publication in peer reviewed journals.

Criterion 9 - Key performance results:

9b   *Key performance indicators: (Indicators used to monitor, understand, predict and understand those outcomes)*

eg   *Percentage of patients in clinically appropriate beds.*
Length of stay.
Number of research projects completed each year.

Criterion 6,7 & 8 - Key measures of stakeholder perception of results:

6,7,8a   *Perception measures: (Direct measures of stakeholder perceptions of the organisation and its results)*
eg: Percentage of patients satisfied with their treatment
Percentage of staff satisfied that they are able
to provide clinically appropriate care for their patients
HSE audit of satisfaction with compliance with
Health and Safety legislation.

Criterion 6,7 & 8 - Key measures of stakeholder perception of results:

6,7,8b   *Perception indicators: (Indicators used to monitor, understand, predict and understand the above levels of satisfaction)*
eg: Achievement of Charter Standards
Rate of complaints/litigation
Sickness and absence rates.

Criterion 1,2,3,4 & 5 - Enablers:

For each sub-criterion part, the approaches used need to be specified.
For example: 1b Leaders are personally involved in ensuring the organisation's management system is developed, implemented and continuously improved.

Approach:

 EFQM self-assessment and review

Degree of Deployment of the Approach to its potential:
Percentage of clinical and managerial leadership staff participating in the approach.

Measured effectiveness:
Number of points achieved by the organisation.

Improvements made:

1997 = 200 points, 1998 = 320 points 1999 = 410 points

Links to results:
Key performance outcomes, levels of stakeholder satisfaction

Criterion 1,2,3,4 & 5 - Enablers (example 2)

Sub-criteria: 5d Products and Services are produced, delivered and serviced:
Approach:

Pre-operative assessment clinics

Degree of Deployment of the Approach to its potential:

Percentage of appropriate surgical specialities using the approach.

Measured effectiveness:

Average length of stay

Improvements made:

1997 = 4 days, 1998 = 3 days 1999 = 2 days

Links to results:

Peri-operative mortality rates, Total FCE's, Income expenditure variance.

1.38   EFQM Reviews 1999 - 2000

Executive Directors generally applied the self-assessment and review process within their departments. They were responsible extensively for this and in many ways turned their local self-assessment and review process into the way they managed their services.

General Managers on the other hand deployed the process invariably. This was partly through the rapidly changing external demands for specific performance outcomes and the day to day crises which typically occured in any complex health care system. In addition, General Managers tended to move on more rapidly and new general managers had to go through a steep learning curve. Very often they took time to become convinced that the process was worthwhile. The most effective general managers made time to train their staff and involve them in the process of self-assessment, review and business planning. Others tended to carry out the process almost mechanistically, prior to the Chief Executive reviews.

However, the Chief Executive Review process now clearly makes high level performance visible and problem areas more easy to detect. This is still uncomfortable for some. The Chief Executive review guidelines have also been further developed to improve the focus on key results and processes and a more effective use of the review time.

Given these outcomes, the purpose of the Chief Executive Review has been further clarified, so as to:

- *recognise good management practices and performance*
- *ensure that actions are focused on Trust priorities*
- *ensure that Trust priorities are relevant and appropriate to the views of the Trust's staff*
- *identify constraints which may affect the achievement of Trust priorities*
- *agree actions and time-scales by which constraints can be removed.*

Executive Directors and General Managers are now expected to ensure that their updated EFQM Self-assessment is sent to the Chief Executive and Excellence Development Director, no later than 10 days before the planned review date.

At the review, the self-assessment team has to present their self-assessment with reference to Trust priorities highlighted on the Self-assessment form and when doing this have to address the following:

Improvement trends for each of the key Trust result areas for which the Executive Director/General Manager has responsibility for. This should be in tabular or graphic format.

Highlight key approaches being used to enable continuous improvement in the key result areas.

Areas of concern in each of the key Trust result areas.

Highlight key approaches which are planned/proposed to be implemented in order to improve performance of key Trust result areas.

Highlight progress and methods of ensuring that EFQM self-assessment and review is fully deployed with the Executive Directors/General Managers area of responsibility.

Issues for guidance, support, clarification etc. (including training and coaching needs) and issues for action by the Chief Executive, Management Board or Trust Board (ie outside of the control of the Executive Director/General Manager's control), should be raised during the presentation on the particular result area of concern.

1.39   Some summary conclusions on Salford's experience

As is obvious from the preceeding account, the EFQM Excellence Model is now well embedded at Salford. The primary aim of implementing the EFQM model and its constituent processes, was that of developing a culture of excellence within a large NHS teaching hospital. Our expereince to date makes obvious that some approaches have worked well, others not as well as expected, but more importantly, a number of key lessons have been learnt.

1.40   Key lessons

The Model has provided clarity as to what the Trust is trying to achieve and has been able to encompass all the new initiatives, which have been imposed on the Trust from outside. This clarity has helped to focus energy on the objectives and targets that the Trust is committed to reaching, in spite of the many changing demands and priorities impacting on the Trust from all sides. Significant change management is known to flounder as time goes on, because the organisation forgets what it was trying to achieve. The clarity as to what the organisation has set out to achieve is provided by the EFQM excellence Model. This has helped to ensure that when new senior managers replace previous managers, any slippage in progress towards that destination of excellence is quickly made visible and corrected. This isn't that simple and straight forward though; some managers still need convincing and still start their new role fire fighting for a while.

In addition, the Trust's own strengths and areas for improvement are now clearly visible, as are the effectiveness of improvement efforts.

However, what the Model does not replace is the leadership and actions which are required to make a difference, in performance. The plan to implement the process of EFQM self-assessment and review top down rather than bottom up, as was the case with the previous TQM process, provided some important successes, but also some key lessons and challenges.

1.41 First time Successes

On the success side, there was from the inception to the present, active participation and commitment to the whole process. It is led by the Chief Executive and the Executive Directors with full support and enthusiasm from the whole of the Trust Board. There are also many front line managers and clinicians who adopted the approach, because they could see its intrinsic value in structuring their approach to continuous improvement which they had started in the days of TQM. These have continued to find ways of improving their services and in sharing good practice with others through the Trust's quality award scheme. Over 160 significant improvements to the service can be demonstrated through these improvement activities and they have continued strongly over the last five years.

1.42 Successes attained following initial failures

However, not all managers and clinicians have made the same level of commitment to EFQM or the process of continual improvement. There are also a few who actively oppose the process, usually by not using the process to review the staff within their area of managerial responsibility. Some do this because they are unable to manage the large demands on their time and resort to fire fighting, rather than managing. Others have not been given enough support to effectively use the approach, not because of lack of training funds, but because of the lack of people, skilled in the EFQM process and its associated management skills of coaching, facilitation and support. The result has been a painful action learning process during which skills have been acquired through trial and error. There are also a few clinicians and manager who oppose the process of involving staff and making performance visible, because they feel it threatens them in some way.

The top down approach adopted in Salford and the time taken to ensure the top team understands what the EFQM Model of Excellence is and how to use the self-assessment and review process, has meant that such threats to the change management process have not been overwhelming. Of particular importance was the early integration of the EFQM process into the normal management processes, rather than parallel to it, as was the case with the TQM process.

However, the main focus of the change management process has been on changing the ethos and value system, rather than on meeting key improvement priorities. To some extent this has been because clinicians and managers are cynical about some of the performance targets imposed on them by national policies, while key resources to achieve improved clinical performance have not been forthcoming. There is a real danger with this. The balance between working on what is important, such as developing measures of clinical performance so as to improve outcomes of treatment and care, can outweigh the need to satisfy the requirement of funding bodies, with their focus on key activity targets.

It should be possible to achieve both within the Model, without losing focus on developing ownership and the culture required.

Although the Trust did not have the resources to allocate significant amounts to the Training required to achieve its ambitious change management program, this was not the primary inhibitor to rapid implementation. Staff who wanted to be trained in the process, all received it. The real factor was the time and priority which staff gave to such training. This can best be seen by the distribution of attendance at training. Staff would attend training if their local managers considered it important enough. However, it should also be recognised that releasing staff for training within the tight staffing levels within the health service is not easy.

Of critical importance was the achievement of commitment by senior managers and particularly clinicians, as the critical factor on sustained and effective change. Consultant clinicians in particular are the key because of two reasons. The first is that they lead the treatment process and determine its priorities and its resource utilisation. Secondly, they are the most stable part of the workforce. Involvement by them results in more long term change, than it does with line managers.

However, clinicians tend to need other clinicians to provide them with leadership and also have difficulty with management concepts which they are not familiar. The management language of the Model thus needs to be carefully reworded to reflect clinical concepts and values, and is better delivered by a fellow clinician. However, clinicians can also be the quickest and the smartest users of the Model. They particularly like the way it has a balanced set of results which includes clinical results, which they see as being particularly missing from NHS management priorities to-date.

Another factor which was revealed slowly was how inadequately clinicians and managers were trained in basic management skills. Few understood process management, process improvement methodologies, problem solving, action planning and effective change management. Many also did not understand the nature of performance indicators and how to interpret these to assess whether they were in line with achieving desired goals or not. Fundamentally, few had really clarified what the results were that they were trying to achieve, as opposed to activities which they were expected to carry out. The self-assessment and review process made these skill gaps visible and resulted in some discussing the merits of the Model, rather than what the Model had revealed about their skills and performance.

Clearly, these skill gaps cannot be filled quickly and the need for a skilled person to identify the development and training needs became increasingly evident as the process of self-assessment progressed. Though the Trust had an Excellence Development Director whose role was to support the Chief Executive in the implementation of the EFQM process, it was not possible for him to also adequately support all the managers and clinicians involved in the next level of the management process. The Trust has now appointed an Excellence Development Facilitator to fill this gap, whose primary role is to support and develop the skills needed by operational clinicians and managers to manage well, within the framework of excellence provided by the Model.

Overall however, the approach used in Salford has gained a life of its own. The effort to involve all staff and to strengthen the approach to improve the overall performance of the Trust shows no sign of weakening. In fact, the commitment and participation rates across the Trust continue to show a significant positive trend.

Case Study 2

South Tees Acute Hospitals NHS Trust (STAHT)

Developing Excellence

2.1 Introduction

In the first case study, the importance of top down involvement and investment in the use of the EFQM Excellence Model was amply demonstrated. Indeed it was a theme that pervaded the whole of the case study. It is a lesson worthy of note and a key message for other organisations embarking on the use of the Excellence model. We would like to reinforce this point and indeed stress the value of senior management involvement, commitment and expertise at integrating the use of the model as an every day management experience. We feel strongly about this and would therefore begin our case study with a view from the very top. We would therefore let Bill Murray OBE, our Chief Executive set the scene and provide a foreword to our case study.

"South Tees Acute Hospitals NHS Trust can be justly proud of its achievements. Since taking on Trust status in 1992, our staff have worked hard to achieve some major local, national and international awards. We already live a culture where our staff are intent to put both themselves and the Trust on the health care map".

"Why introduce the EFQM Excellence Model? Modern health care is ever changing. The demand for services and improvements to patient care, as well as being financially responsible, continue to challenge us. Our move to a single hospital in 2003 means we have to look systematically at everything we do. If we are to continue to provide excellent health care, we need to look closely at where we are, where we would like to be and how we are planning to get there. In many ways the advent of the single site hospital has concentrated our minds. We have a momentous event on the near horizon. What is important at this time is planning our way to this event".

"This is where the EFQM Excellence Model comes into the picture. It provides us with a framework for continuous improvement. Not just a quick fix. It is a long term project, which may never reach a conclusion. What it provides us with is a new way of working, a new culture, to integrate into our already very 'go for it' way of life. For the first time we have a tangible way of establishing baselines, setting targets and monitoring results. These results then become our new baselines, and we can set new targets. What difference does this make to patients? Our patients are already seeing a difference and will continue to see significant changes in the way we provide our service".

"The main strength of the Excellence Model is that it allows staff from different functions to work together to improve services. In our quest to become the best single site hospital in Europe, we need more than ever before to design our care around our patients. I believe we have, in the Excellence Model, the tools to do just that and meet the challenges of delivering excellent modern health care".

Bill Murray

2.2   Background

The South Tees Acute Hospitals NHS Trust (STAHT) is based in Middlesbrough and provides health care from three main sites. STAHT was established in April 1992, and provides both district general hospital and tertiary services. The area STAHT serves is recognised nationally, both in economic and health terms, as one of the poorest in the country. Mortality rates are high and approximately one third of these deaths are attributable to heart disease. An equal number are caused by cancer, particularly lung cancer. STAHT employs almost 5000 staff and has a budget of £174.000,000. During the 1999/00 period, they provided treatment and care to 107,987 inpatients and day cases, 268,899 outpatients and treated 80,780 accident and emergency cases.

One of the major aims for STAHT since its inception, has been the drive to provide all of its services from a single site. STAHT has signed an agreement with a consortium, to fund this development through the Government's Private Finance Initiative. Construction commenced in August 1999, with completion due within 44 months. Our new hospital will provide a "state of the art" environment, which will enable first class health care services to be delivered. Inter site transfers will be eradicated. It will support excellent clinical relationships by ensuring physical proximity, a luxury we have not experienced to date.

2.3   Organisational structure

The organisational structure within STAHT centres around a mechanism to support a direct relationship between the patient and the consultant, i.e. a clinical speciality. Specialities are grouped together to form a clinical directorate. 34 clinical directorates are grouped to form 10 clinical divisions. The Clinical Divisions operate as semi-autonomous 'business' units, with devolved authority and decision making. The Trust Board and Management Group provide the overall direction and guidance by setting organisational objectives, with the Divisions having flexibility at implementation.

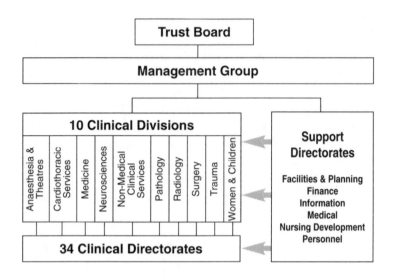

Fig. 1 Structure of the South Tees Acute Hospitals NHS Trust

The structure emphasises the key role that clinicians play in providing health services and they are actively involved in the management of the organisation. STAHT has been nationally recognised as an exemplar site for their model of "clinicians in management". Out of the 18 members of the management group, 14 are from a clinical background, and 12 of them are consultants.

2.4   History of quality improvement at STAHT

In the late 1980's, the then hospital units were actively involved in district wide initiatives such as the 'Patient Perception Group', 'Putting People First', and the production of a 'Guide to Good Practice'. In 1989, the hospital units and health authority, led by Bill Murray, the then Director of Planning for the Health Authority, became a National Demonstration Site for Total Quality Management (TQM). This involved the application of 'industrial' concepts and principles of TQM into a NHS organisation. This approach provided many benefits to STAHT. Primarily, it led to the development of a quality culture with over 10 years achievement and recognition. In addition, STAHT has successfully achieved positive clinical leadership through the integration of doctors in management and a devolved approach to managing clinical teams. Several quality initiatives including Patient Centred Care, Quality

Circles, Clinical Audit and the development of STAHT Core Values, were implemented, with varying degrees of success. All of Facilities Management (catering, laundry etc.) and the Radiotherapy department are accredited to ISO 9002. Though beneficial in their respective ways, a review of the respective approaches not surprisingly, made obvious the perception that they were seen as a fragmented group of separate initiatives and not part of a co-ordinated approach to continuous quality improvement. To some, there was a sense that the initiatives were very much 'flavour of the month' and led to 'initiative overload'. (See Fig. 2)

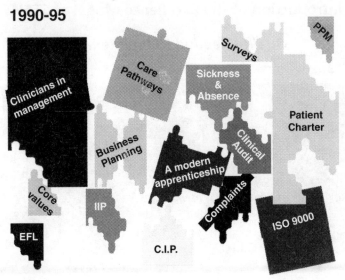

Fig. 2 Fragmented approach to quality improvement-like pieces of an incomplete jigsaw

What was required was an over-arching framework that could be used to develop an integrated approach to achieving significant improvement in the delivery of health care, across the whole organisation. This needed to be achieved through positive clinical leadership and through the involvement of multi-professional/multi-agency staff, working together in reviewing and redesigning processes. And like all other NHS Trusts, we also wanted to focus more on direct achievements and results. Moreover, we wanted an approach which could sustain performance and quality of service in tandem.

In 1995, the Chief Executive became interested in the European Foundation for Quality Management (EFQM) Excellence Model. The Excellence Model was seen as a mechanism to build upon all of the previous quality improvement work and integrate them as normal day to day operations. STAHT called this approach:

"Developing Excellence"

2.5   Introduction of the Excellence Model at STAHT

Quality needed to be integrated

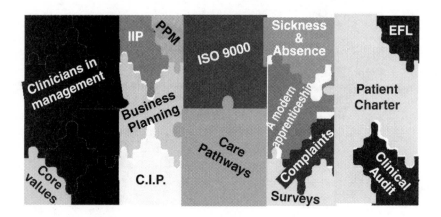

Fig. 3 Developing Excellence - an integrated approach

The rationale for an integrated and coherent framework was outlined earlier. We now wish to provide an outline on the manner in which we introduced the model at STAHT.

In 1994, there was both a perception and desire for STAHT to operate in a fundamentally different way. As we mentioned earlier, there was a fragmented approach to quality improvement. Additionally, there was a drive to achieve the major strategic development to provide all services from a single site. The ultimate aim was to a become a Centre of Excellence providing Patient

Centred Care. Whilst improving quality has always been the main driver for STAHT, there was also a parallel realisation and a convincing business case, that a single site development could realise significant revenue savings. Any approach that STAHT were to pursue, would therefore need to be patient centred and improve quality, but equally reduce costs.

A Management Consultant (SDC Partnership), introduced the Excellence Model to the Chief Executive, Bill Murray, in the autumn of 1994. It was promoted as a framework for implementing and managing the overall strategy, integrating all previous approaches to improvement, promoting patient centred care, as well as offering a mechanism through which business case economies could be achieved.

Up until 1994, the EFQM model had only been adopted in the private sector. Plans to introduce the model into the public sector in 1995 were afoot, but at that time there was no blue print as to how the model could be applied to health care. A major deciding factor for STAHT was the fact that the Excellence Model provided a framework for self assessment. The process offered a comprehensive, systematic and integrated framework by which STAHTs as an organisation could assess, measure and review its activities and results against each of the nine criteria of the model. Furthermore, the model fostered the use of enabling improvement strategies and plans, as the basis of regular review of progress towards the agreed objectives. It was generally felt that the model would enable:

- *a rigorous and structured approach to Patient centred care*
- *an assessment based on fact and not individual perception*
- *a means to achieve consistency of direction and consensus on what needs to be done*
- *a way to ensure people meaningfully apply the principles on excellence*
- *a means to create enthusiasm amongst all staff and give fresh impetus to their pursuit of excellence*
- *a means of measuring progress over time*
- *a means to benchmark, both internally and against other organisations across Europe.*

2.6 Self Assessment - South Tees approach

A number of commentators have suggested that the EFQM model could be adopted in a variety of ways. Our starting point was through self assessment and the manner in which we pursued this was to pilot it in a couple of areas and then assess the benefits. Throughout 1995, three separate areas carried out self assessments and produced action plans to address areas for improvement.

The first, the Directorate of General Surgery, was about to embark on major change. The Directorates' wards were spread over two hospital sites and they were moving, as part of site rationalisation, onto one site. The focus of the move was patient centred care and therefore the Directorate was keen to pilot a mechanism that would help them achieve their goal.

The approach used, with guidance and support from SDC Partnership, was as follows:

- *Select the self assessment review team*
  This included the Divisional Manager, the Clinical Manager and a Ward Sister from the Directorate of Surgery. The rest of the team included the Director of Personnel, who was to lead "Developing Excellence", and the six members of the Quality and Organisation Development team.

- *Educate and train the self-assessment team asassessors.*
  The team took four days out, with three days training as assessors using the standard case study approach.

- *Determine the assessment tasks and actions required for each element of the framework.*
  Each team member was assigned criteria and had to gather the evidence relating to the Directorate for that criterion part. This involved interviews, focus groups and document gathering.

- **Conduct the self-assessment**
An assessment document was produced, assessed individually and then the team met to agree the main strengths, areas for improvement, and the score.

- **Determine the immediate action plan**
A report was produced with recommendations for action.

- **Setting up the improvement teams/actions to implement the action plan**
This also involved identifying a Project Manager to co-ordinate and lead the various project teams.

The first assessment created increasing interest around the Trust. The pilot was extended to a couple of other interested areas. One was the Division of Women and Children, which comprised four Directorates, Obstetrics, Gynaecology, Paediatrics and Neonatology. The other area was largely a non-clinical area, the Directorate of Information. These two pilot areas followed the same process described above.

The Director of Personnel and leader for Developing Excellence, briefed Senior Managers as follows:

"Quality means improving everything we do though involving all the people within the organisation. Awards such as ISO 9000 are a measure of the systems and processes we have in place, while Standards such as Investor in People focus on communication, training and development. None of them on their own gives a total picture of what we're doing to become a quality organisation".

"At its simplest, this quality model asserts that if you have the right people working in the right way, you get the right results."

"Excellence doesn't mean the quality work we've already done is wasted. On the contrary, it builds on the work we've already done. You can see on the model where all the awards and accreditation fit in. We should be using the Model to achieve quality".

2.7   Some early lessons learnt

Even at an early stage of working with the Model, it became apparent that a number of key lessons were emerging and we would like to reflect on these in terms of the actions we adopted at addressing them. They include 3 key lessons as follows:

- *The language at the time was very alien to clinical staff.*
Our action and advice was to change the language to one that is familiar to the staff group and the organisation. For example we used the term 'patient' rather than 'customer', and 'clinical outcomes' rather than business results.

- *Involvement of medical staff from the beginning is crucial.*
The Division of Women and Children included four medical staff in the assessor training and the assessment process. They were the Chief of Service, a Clinical Director and two consultants. This tactic had the effect of greater commitment to the change agenda.

- *Keep the action plan to a manageable size.*
The first pilot, in their enthusiasm, initially attempted to tackle too many areas for improvement. We now ensure that actions are prioritised and limited to a number that one can handle.

By the end of 1995, some of the early concerns that the Excellence Model was going to be very prescriptive and a little like "dot to dot", management were being dispelled. There was now a ground swell of opinion that the Model was applicable to health care and could benefit patients as well as the organisation. It was now time to attempt a corporate assessment.

2.8   Corporate self assessments

Early in January 1996, the management group attended a two day workshop facilitated by the Management Consultants. The group performed the first corporate assessment using their observations, as well as some of the evidence from the pilot areas. STAHT has since performed two other corporate assessments. The second assessment, used Teamscore, a computer based method, and involved the Developing Excellence Steering Group in gathering the relevant evidence. The third assessment, in 1999, used an award style process with a submission type document. The document was assessed individually by a team of 5 trained internal assessors (including 2 senior managers) and two experienced external assessors. STAHT as well as one of its Divisions have now made a submission for the Excellence North East Award 2000. This will provide an external assessment of achievement and the results of this are expected in November 2000.

The individual Divisions have also performed self-assessments using different methods. They range from a questionnaire-based survey, facilitated workshop through to an award simulation approach. Based on experience, we have found that all methods of self-assessment are useful. There is no one right way. In selecting an approach though, an organisation will need to consider the implications of the alternatives in terms of time, cost and quality of output. The primary purpose of undertaking self-assessment is to drive continuous improvement. It provides a picture of the status of the organisation, usually in terms of strengths, areas for improvement and sometimes a score.

An award simulation self-assessment based on available evidence will provide a more accurate score. The downside to this is that the demand made on staff and time are considerable. For a corporate assessment, this investment in time may well be justified. The other methods of self-assessment will provide reasonable information and useful outcomes. It should however be acknowledged that accuracy and validity does decrease with the reduction in people and time commitment. We have found that other methods are extremely useful at Divisional, Directorate level or team level.

2.9 What we found

The first corporate assessment demonstrated many areas for improvement. We thought we were good. In NHS terms we delivered what was expected of us. We had met all of our financial targets and we had achieved local, national and international awards. It was rather sobering to discover that we had only scored a grand total of 217 points out of a possible 1000! (Top European companies score 700). The priority areas for improvement were within **Leadership, People Management, Processes, Customer, People and Business Results (now known as Key Performance Results).**

The Director of Personnel was assigned to lead 'Developing Excellence'. Senior Managers and Clinical Leaders either expressed an interest or were approached to lead a specific project area for improvement. These people became known as the Developing Excellence Steering Group. The Chief Executive has been an active member of the Developing Excellence Steering Group since the outset. The membership of the group has been reviewed annually at the end of the year. Membership has now increased to include the Chairman of the Trust Board and 3 non- Executive Board members. More than half the Management Group and all the Divisional Managers have been involved in one or more of the project groups.

The Developing Excellence Steering Group

Chief Executive
Director of Personnel (Chair until retired in January 1999)
Director of Organisation Development (Chair from January 1999)
Director of Finance (Current Chair)
Chairman and 3 Non Executive Directors
Director of Nursing Development (Lead, Partnership working)
Medical Director
Director of Facilities and Planning (Lead, Policy and Strategy)
Chief of Service, Cardiothoracic Services,(Lead, Customer and Staff Satisfaction Steering Group)
Chief of Service, Non Medical Clinical Services, Acting Director of Information (Leadership and Key Performance results Steering Group)
Clinical Director Obstetrics, Lead, Obstetric project.
Director of the Learning Alliance, Northern and Yorkshire, (Process Redesign and Process Leadership)
Divisional Manager, Radiology, (Deputy lead, Customer and staff Satisfaction Steering Group)
Divisional Manager, Medicine, (Lead, Processes Steering Group)
Divisional Manager, Surgery
Divisional Finance Manager
Director of Cancer Services Development.

The Developing Excellence Steering Group meets monthly to agree priorities for corporate improvement activities and associated funding. They also monitor and review progress. Reports are then made to the Management Group and the Trust Board on a quarterly basis. The annual review day for the Developing Excellence involves an update of progress from all the development activities, a review of the overall approach taken and the planning of next year's agenda. Recommendations are presented to the Management Group and then to the Divisional Managers, who ensure they are acted upon.

It is now generally recognised that the Developing Excellence Steering Group has almost fulfilled its remit. Given that its membership is coterminous with the Management Group, it has been decided that the latter group will take the lead and steer Developing Excellence, during 2001 and onwards.

2.10. Developing Excellence: Actions and achievements

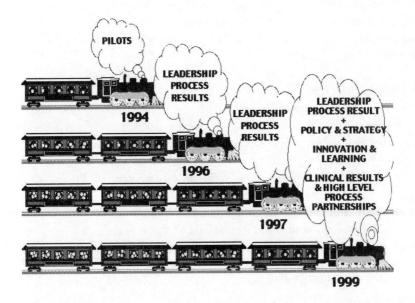

Fig. 4. Our Journey to Excellence.

We have earlier touched upon the reasons as to why we began this journey and how we approached it. Now we need to reflect upon actions and achievements. As is obvious in Fig. 4 , ours was an incremental approach, focusing on a few key elements at first, and then gradually increasing and widening our focus as momentum developed as is outlined in Fig. 4. 'Our Journey to Excellence'. Our main emphasis initially was, Leadership, Processes and Results. Each year, through demonstrating successes, more issues and more staff came 'on board'. We would now like to describe some of the issues, processes and outcomes of each of these projects. First though some details on the Leadership project.

2.11   Leadership

Raising the standards of leadership within STAHT was identified as one of the key areas for improvement. The Leadership Project Steering Group first met in March 1996. The members were senior managers, including two medical staff. Bill Murray, the Chief Executive led the project with project management support from the Director of Information.

The self-assessment indicated that whilst we had some very good leaders, this was not universal across the organisation. We had not identified what we expected of leaders. More fundamentally, we had not identified or really understood 'Who are our Leaders'? The remit of the Leadership Project Steering Group was to:

- *clarify those with leadership roles by*
  define what we mean by leadership;
  identifying who does what;
  assessing who the key staff groups look to for leadership.

- *Assess Leadership Management Skills and Competencies*
  define leadership competencies and skills;
  set minimum standards for leaders;
  implement mechanism to audit compliance with standards;
  identify Reward and Recognition Mechanisms;
  research and appraise non- pay reward systems;
  review the strengths and weaknesses of the existing "Thank you awards";
  establish a sub group to take this forward.

There was initially a wide-ranging debate about the meaning of leadership. Key issues raised and subsequently clarified included issues such as:

> *the distinction between a manager and a leader*
> *concepts such as vision and charisma*
> *the importance of technical excellence as a selection criteria*
> *the need to ensure that innovation is encouraged.*

Each Division and Directorate categorised all those who held leadership positions. Fundamentally the category consisted of all managers and those in a position of influence and included Consultants, Ward Managers as well as Corporate Directors and Clinical Directors.

A member of the group carried out a detailed analysis on management competencies related to leadership roles. At the end of 1997, the group had identified and agreed what they initially described as minimum leadership standards. These statements were considered to be very basic standards. They were intended to clarify for those in leadership positions, the key elements of effective leadership consistent with STAHT's core values.

It was originally proposed to carry out a centrally co-ordinated 'audit' to determine where these standards were not being achieved. This was not however favourably received. Concerns were expressed regarding the bureaucracy and inspection elements, which did not fit well with the organisation's culture. The management group eventually agreed that the standards would be introduced, that they would be referred to as Minimum People Standards, and that compliance would be assessed during the Positive Performance Management appraisals.

2.12 Leadership development programme

In addition, the Leadership Project Steering group agreed that a developmental approach would be taken to enhancing leadership. The emphasis was placed on role clarification, self assessment and providing development opportunities. Members of the steering group considered the 360° appraisal instruments available and with support from a management consultant, introduced the Leadership Effectiveness Analysis (LEA) Questionnaire, as the assessment part of a Leadership Development Programme.

The LEA is an appraisal questionnaire, which is based upon 6 functions of leadership and 22 leadership behaviours. The 6 Leadership functions are:

Creating a Vision
Developing Followers
Implementing the Vision
Following Through
Achieving Results
Team Playing.

Each of the functions is broken down into behaviours. For example:

- Creating a Vision can be seen to encompass elements of behaviour which are characterised by:
    - *being Traditional*
    - *promoting Innovation*
    - *being Technical*
    - *decision making by Self*
    - *being Strategic.*

The LEA can be used for self analysis or as a 360° appraisal tool. 360° appraisal was successfully piloted with a group of interested Clinical Directors. So far all the Chiefs of Service, the Corporate Directors, the Divisional Managers, 37 out of 39 Clinical Directors and all of the Process Leaders have taken part in the Leadership Development Programme which starts with the LEA. In total, some 320 leaders have embarked on the Leadership Development Programme.

The 360° appraisal process involves the individual filling in a self completed questionnaire, then asking 3 peers, 3 people that report directly to them and their 'boss' to fill in the questionnaire. The completed questionnaires are sent away for analysis. A trained internal assessor then gives confidential feedback to the individual. Each individual is offered mentoring and one to one coaching support. The majority of LEAs have been done with groups of staff and has resulted in customised leadership programmes being developed to address common knowledge and skill requirements.

Whole divisional management teams have undergone the leadership development programme together. The majority of whom have shared their individual profiles. This indicates that strong working relationships have developed between Managers and Consultants. The Leadership Development Programme also involves clarifying future roles and identifying future behavioural competencies. This then gives participants an idea of their development needs.

2.13 Organisational characteristics

We have also been able to consider behaviour profiles common to the Trust. When reviewing group 'self score' behaviour profiles, over 80% scored between 75-99 on EMPATHY, revealing a high degree of sensitivity. The basic desire to help, care and being sensitive to helping others is firmly embedded in our people. Over 60% (and over 85% of clinicians) scored between 80-99 on the TRADITIONAL scale. This is understandable as the approach to delivering care is based on experience. A TRADITIONAL approach values the teaching of experience. Viewing the past as a determinant of the future is firmly held, particularly by clinicians. This may however lead to ideas and novel initiatives being rejected, simply because they are new and untested.

COMMUNICATING and DELEGATING are highly valued both from a business and clinical viewpoint. People are given the information and left to get on with delivering the tasks. There are very few control mechanisms exerted on people. People are trusted to deliver. Finally, TECHNICAL in depth analysis is a preferred approach to problem solving.

2.14 Organisational implications

In order for STAHT to deliver it's future policy and strategy, it clearly needed to build upon the existing leadership strengths in terms of core leadership behaviour, but also to balance them with skills and values. The strong emphases on TRADITIONAL and TECHNICAL behaviours need to be balanced with additional emphasis on INNOVATION. Unless this is addressed, opportunities for new approaches, harnessing creative energy of the whole organisation may be lost as people emphasise the importance of experience. Approaches may be lost because they are new and untried. Furthermore, an emphasis on COMMUNICATION and DELEGATION can lead to empowerment when you have competent people. Balancing these two behaviours with PERSUASION (to engage people) and FEEDBACK (to ensure trust and delivery), can enable an organisation to move forward with energy, trust and commitment.

Similarly, CONSENSUAL behaviour counterbalances the desire to fight one's corner. Whilst each leadership group, chiefs of service, corporate directors, and divisional managers etc. have all identified key future leadership behaviours which vary according to role, certain core elements of attributes such as PERSUASION, FEEDBACK and CONSENSUAL, were seen to be common to all of the groups.

2.15   General benefits to date.

So what have we achieved on this front. Formal evaluation through individual feedback forms and observed change by others, has identified the following positive outcomes:

-clarity of roles and required behaviours with renewed enthusiasm and energy for such roles
-team building and development
-identified individual development plans which link into organisation, clinical and business developments e.g. Clinical Governance
-sharing of profiles between managers and clinicians, which we believe is unique within the NHS. The benefit being that they are able to complement each others strengths, and minimise potential liabilities.

The staff satisfaction survey has also been used to evaluate the effectiveness of the Leadership Development Programme. For instance, there has been a 7% increase in staff who feel valued by their manager and an overall increase in the leadership associated results. All Divisional Managers and 50% of the Corporate Directors are mentors to other Leaders within the Trust. There are now plans to increase the number of mentors across the Trust.

General patterns and trends are useful in themselves, but what about specific cases of outcomes reflecting such developments. As a case in point, collaborative efforts between the Clinical Director for Oral Surgery and Orthodontics and the Lead Cancer Clinician for ENT, have led to a multi-agency team in the review of Head, Neck and Oral systems and processes. Similarly, the Chief of Service for the Division of Medicine has led a reconfiguration of services that has resulted in an 8% increase in patients treated, a 12% reduction in bed day occupancy and reduced the average length of stay to 1.5 days.

2.16   Some lessons learnt

Overall, our experience in managing this part of implementation of Developing Excellence has indicated that:

- *it takes time - longer than anticipated*
- *there is a need to manage people's expectations*
- *it requires ongoing investment*
- *there is a need for external consultant support in the early days*
- *top level support and commitment, from the Chief Executive, Medical Director remains crucial*
- *individual coaching/mentoring makes a huge difference to establishing behavioural change.*

2.17   Reward and recognition mechanisms

The Leadership Steering Group also carried out a major review of non-pay reward and recognition in 1996. Their findings were implemented in 1997/1998. They reviewed the then current recognition systems through an internal survey and also conducted research into what happens in other organisations, both in the public and the private sector. The survey demonstrated that whilst recipients of a Thank You Award were generally satisfied with the type of reward, i.e. a voucher, it was not always timely. The Chairman at a special ceremony used to present the thank you awards, 2 or 3 times a year. It was found that 48% of staff were not aware of the scheme. Furthermore, a small minority of staff felt that the awards were 'lukewarm' gestures, which singled out employees and departments whilst alienating others and above all, were soon forgotten.

As a result of the above the group made a number of recommendations which have now been implemented. They include:

- *Encouraging a climate of recognition.*

This has resulted in a number of small but more inclusive surprises. For instance, the Chief of Service and Divisional Manager for the Division of Medicine presented a "crème egg" at Easter to all their staff. They were delivered to the wards and departments in small Easter baskets. At Christmas each team and ward in the Women and Children Division received a box of chocolates from the Divisional

Manager. This Divisional Manager also recently sent flowers to 3 members of staff who had to deal with a very distressing situation.

- **Improved Thank You Award Scheme.**

Communication regarding the Thank You Award has been increased with posters and leaflets displayed around the hospitals. The awards are presented in a more timely manner at the ward or department. The Chairman or a non-executive member of the Trust Board presents the awards monthly. There have been 22 thank you awards presented this year so far. These have included nominations from line managers and patients.

- **Long service award**

The Trust Board agreed to a long service award and this was introduced in January 1999. Staff who have 25 years service within the NHS are entitled to 4 weeks additional annual leave non-recurringly. This leave can be taken any time, service permitting, either all together or as separate weeks.

- **Trust Team of the Year Award**

The Chief Executive launched the first Team of the Year Award in 1998 as a method of encouraging, recognising and rewarding the improvement activity at ward and department level. To date, the Trust has been fortunate in receiving sponsorship for the scheme.

To be eligible for the award, projects must demonstrate that they have led to an improvement in the service provided. Projects directly supervised by senior managers are excluded. The purpose for the award is to reward local, not corporate projects. Each of the shortlisted project teams and the overall winner, receive a monetary prize and attend an award dinner and disco at the Cellnet Riverside Stadium. For two years, there has also been an award for the best Clinical Audit project, sponsored by Janssen-Cilag.

We have discussed in some detail, systems and mechanisms for addressing the Leadership dimension and to some extent enabling issues relating to people development and reward and recognition. We now want to turn to the issue of process development.

2.18   Becoming a 'process' centred health care organisation.

The use of the EFQM as a conceptual model for developing organisational effectiveness has led STAHT to develop its approach at process redesign within the overall framework. Two factors within the Excellence Model have influenced our approach to redesign. These are the wide range of results and the critical linkage between process and leadership. Both factors are now discussed.

During the early self assessments, we quickly realised that we knew very little about processes and how to become a process centred organisation. The first point of analysis was to understand Business Process Re-engineering (BPR) approaches. Like others, we made recourse to the literature produced by *Hammer and Champy (1994) and the many others who have contributed to the BPR debate.

The essence of the BPR methodology appeared relevant to our desired organisational outcomes. BPR purports to enable the organisation to increase the speed and quality of service provision, an aspect that was of central importance to STAHT. However, other elements of the methodology appeared to be in conflict with our own core values, the principles of excellence and the current reality of health care delivery.

The well documented failure rates of 70% for BPR projects worried the Developing Excellence Steering Group. We could not sustain a failure rate of 70%. Additionally, the focus upon cost-reduction was not something we believed should be an explicit project outcome. It was clear that NHS staff were unlikely to engage in the pursuit of change if they believed the methodology to be focused solely upon cost reduction.

The final influencing factor was the methodological assumptions about the development of generalist versus specialist roles. Current realities in health care are driving us towards on the one hand to more specialisation, whereas on the other, we are witnessing the development of hybrid professional roles (nurse consultant, paramedic, specialist GP's). The realisation of the above issues led the steering group to carefully consider how the approach to redesign should be developed. During this time, the team from Leicester Royal Infirmary provided invaluable support. STAHT will always be indebted to them for the honesty they demonstrated when sharing what they had learnt, both good and not so good. Sharing good practice remains one of the enduring aspects of learning within the health service.

2.19 The STAHT approach to designing health care processes

The main focus upon process redesign centred around our desire to deliver on the wide portfolio of results demanded by the Excellence Model. This approach we believed has moved us away from the simplistic approach of BPR, to focus on:

> • Patient/carer satisfaction
> • Delivery of clinically effective care
> • Staff satisfaction
> • Efficient use of resources.

Fig. 5 Excellence Results in Health care used by STAHT

We have developed an approach that is very simple and is based upon 3 key stages.

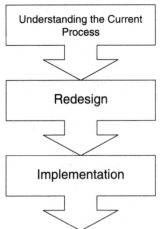

Fig. 6 Stages of Process Redesign

Each Stage has specific aims

A) Understanding the current process

To help the team clarify how their system works

To enable the team to identify key performance (process) problems

To ensure the identification of bottleneck

To understand why improvement efforts have previously failed

To enable to team to measure the degree of improvement achieved.

B) Redesign

To design and process that which delivers the range of results identified in Fig. 5

To ensure patients, not professions are the centre of the patient journey

To design job/roles which deliver the process – not make the process fit the current roles

To strive to achieve step change – but accept incremental change/moves in the right direction.

C) Implementation

To apply principles of rapid cycle improvement - Plan – Test – Learn and Evaluate

To deliver sustainable long term improvements

To build organisational capacity for continuous improvement

To develop a performance framework, which could be managed at the team level; an 8-step model was developed.

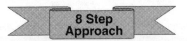

8 Step Approach

- **Identifying the process**
- **Defining the project boundaries**
- **Identifying the project**
- **Understanding the current process**
- **Identifying future process requirements**
- **Creating a vision**
- **Redesign**
- **Implementation and review**

Fig. 7 The 8 steps to process redesign

To underpin the successful delivery of the redesign approach outlined above, key principles have been established as follows:-

Building capacity for good change management is as important as other project outcomes.

To achieve this, a truly bottom up approach has to be developed. We encourage cross-functional teams (a member from each work area who contributes to the delivery of the process) to undertake the project. Our approach denies the idea of using 'the brightest and the best' and is underpinned by the assumption that everyone can contribute to service improvement.

Job security has to be assured if you want to deliver real change.

Fundamental to radically changing service provision is the issue of job security. Step change usually requires the development of alternative roles. Roles, which are designed around patient needs means that previously held roles must change. Staff are unlikely to become energised if they think they may be made redundant. The NHS must truly practice 'staff centred' change, if real benefits are to be achieved. Within STAHT, all staff are assured of their continued employment and current financial reward. What is not assured is the role and function that they will have in the future. Ultimately this will depend upon patient need.

High level project management and facilitation skills are central to success

Busy clinical teams need help to make redesign run smoothly. This type of support is essential if success is to be assured.

Start at the sub process level where it all makes sense.

Building capacity by helping staff to learn the skills to deliver redesign means starting small. Taking on hugely ambitious projects in the early days before the organisation understands the methodology of redesign is a sure way to increase the risk of failure.

2.20   The Link between process centering and leadership

Having established a successful approach to process redesign, the use of the Excellence Model has led us to re-consider the critical link with leadership. It was decided early in our development programme that we would not rush into restructuring around critical processes, unless we had evidence that it would positively impact upon our portfolio of results. The opportunity was used to enhance our current managerial arrangements by becoming oriented to cross-functional processes.

2.20.1   The Challenge

Here however resides some key challenges. How does one really deliver a seamless patient journey, when each step of that journey is functionally managed in separate silos? This issue challenged and exercised the minds of the early teams undertaking redesign at STAHT.

It became obvious that an arrangement had to be made whereby, the performance of the whole process could be continuously improved. But continuously improving a whole patient journey requires several critical issues to be considered:-

- *the overall journey must be understood*
- *the targets for performance must be understood, agreed and owned by all who work along the process*
- *a method of monitoring the process must be established by the team*
- *a means of continuously improving the wide portfolio of results for the process must be established.*

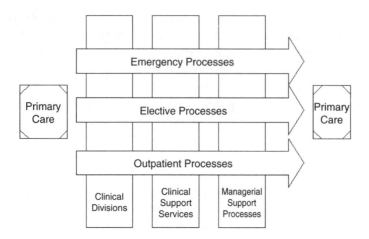

Fig. 8 Key processes which reflects the patients journey cross the main functions.

2.20.2 Establishing real performance management at the level of the patient journey

If the patient journey is to be continuously improved, then the team must own the performance management framework. Performance management at the sub process level makes sense. By understanding how many patients (inputs) are entering the care process and how this relates to planned and target activity levels, the process team were able to act very quickly to changes in activity. It was found that management of performance at this level provides the organisation with an 'early warning system' for shifts in activity.

Monitoring only becomes performance management once the team is able to act, within agreed guidelines, to ensure planned activity levels are achieved. How this is achieved within health care is outside the scope of this case study. However, leaders of health care must address this issue in order to be successful.

Having identified that inputs needed to be monitored and managed, the next important part of the performance framework centres around key cycle times (time between different steps of the process). In health care services, many parts of the patient journey are dependent upon the previous step. The team can't plan treatment interventions without first diagnosing the patient, which requires tests to be completed. Teams need to understand how long each part of the process will take. Only at this point will they be able to smoothly manage patient flows (throughput). When the team understands what has gone on before and what will follow after their process step, they will become more capable of preventing problems, as well as managing actual ones.

Clinical effectiveness needs to be integral to the performance framework. Teams often experience initial difficulty in identifying what must and could be monitored. Often teams set themselves the virtually impossible task of creating a perfect clinical governance framework. Pragmatism and on going development are required in the absence of a National Service framework. Linked to the clinical element of any framework, is the issue of outputs and outcomes.

The process team is perfectly placed to monitor the length of the patient journey. The team monitors how many leave the care process at particular stages and how many continue to receive care at different stages (i.e. on-going out-patient review).

Moving on from the quantitative elements of a performance framework – it must also address with equal vigour the qualitative and in particular, the satisfaction elements of service provision. A summary is provided in Fig. 9

1. **Patients entering care process (in-puts)**
2. **Key cycle times**
3. **Clinical effectiveness indicators**
4. **Patient satisfaction**
5. **Staff satisfaction**
6. **Patients leaving the process of care**

Fig. 9 Elements to be included in a process centred performance management framework

Although this framework may appear simplistic, it has evolved over the period of our work. The learning associated with the evolutionary process made us consider the question, '*how can cross-functional processes be led?*'

2.21   Process leadership

As part of the Trust-wide approach to Leadership Development, we used the LEA 360º appraisal questionnaire to develop our Process Leaders. We have also investigated the development of this emergent role. Our action research has led us to conclude that in addition to functional management, cross-functional process teams need leaders. We believe it is virtually impossible to reshape around a sub process team; we may be proved wrong! Additionally, what ever form (structure) you place around a team, boundaries will always exist. The boundaries may take the form of professional demarcation, or intra-agency cultural difference etc. It occurred to our team, that leaders needed to be able to work and lead across boundaries. This assumption has resulted in the development of our 'Leading Across Boundaries programme'. Process Leaders have worked to identify the behaviours, which they believe to be critical to success. Their experience tells us that:-

- *Leaders must understand (not control) the whole process and the interconnections between all the component steps.*
- *Control is not a feature of process leadership. It is the performance management framework developed by the team, which includes cycle times and quality indicators, that controls the process. Process Leaders support, help and coach Process Step owners to achieve agreed levels of performance.*
- *Process Leaders must be the focus for continuous improvement, inspiring the team to even-higher levels of performance – on behalf of the patient. To achieve, this they need to have well developed creativity skills, the ability to be innovative and to be able to help others to innovate.*
- *The ability to communicate effectively and most importantly provide feedback is crucial. Process leaders work from a position of influence, not managerial power. Providing feedback is often the only means of resolving performance problems.*

The work with leadership and processes continues to evolve. We certainly don't have all the answers; but we have begun to understand the questions. The staff who have embraced redesign as a means of improving patient care have and continue to be, inspirational. The way in which they've redesigned services, which satisfied the results portfolio of the Excellence Model, served as a lesson to us all. The NHS have immensely talented staff; the trick is to develop their skills in redesign and watch them grow.

2.22 Results

The enabling elements of leadership, people, rewards and recognition and processes have so far, commanded much of the attention of the case study. We now want to turn our attention to a discussion of the concept of results. In effect our patients as customers, our people i.e. staff and partners in health care, together with society in general all expect the health services to deliver a quality service. None more so than central government, evidenced through ever increasing targets and expectations of key performance results. In this regard we will discuss some of our strategies and what we have achieved.

2.22.1 Customer results

The Corporate Self-Assessments identified that whilst STAHT had previously carried out patient and GP surveys, very little action was taken as a result. The Customer Satisfaction Steering Group was established and was responsible for planning an approach that would deliver meaningful results. The previous surveys had been managed externally by market research companies. It was thought that if the surveys were managed in-house, there would be more ownership of the results and more action would ensue.

The Customer Satisfaction Steering Group designed a questionnaire during 1997, following a series of Focus Groups interviews, in order to determined what was important to patients. The Trust has since carried out two such surveys.

2.22.2 Patient surveys

The corporate survey deals with common themes such as Information, Communication and Facilities. Individual Directorates are encouraged to perform their own speciality specific surveys, that deal particularly with their specific contexts. The questionnaire asks patients to rate their level of satisfaction, as well as the level of importance, using a Likert scale structured as follows:

Very dissatisfied	Very unimportant
Dissatisfied	Unimportant
Satisfied	Important
Very Satisfied	Very Important

The patient's names and addresses are obtained, over a two month period from the Patient Administration System, following discharge. The questionnaires are sent out to all the patients from that two month period, with an accompanying letter and a pre-paid paid envelope. The response rate has been 52% and 49% respectively. Each Division receives a breakdown of their results and comments, compared with the Trust average.

Following the first survey, the Customer Satisfaction Steering Group recommended that corporate and divisional targets to be included in the business plans. The results displayed in Fig. 10 are those that have corporate targets and those that were rated as "very important" by patients. All of the results with the exception of car parking, show considerable improvement. Car parking will cause some difficulties until building work on the single site has been completed. We have also carried out two outpatient clinics surveys.

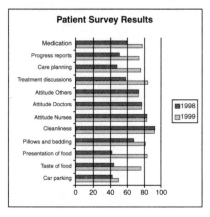

Fig. 10 A sample of the Patient Survey Results

2.22.3 The GP survey

The Chair of the Customer Satisfaction Steering Group initially met with a group of GPs to establish what was important to them. The questions were then grouped around these areas. The Trust then carried out a survey in December 1998, using a format similar to that of the patient survey, in that it asked about level of importance as well as satisfaction. The main area of "dissatisfaction" was around discharge with clarity of discharge letters rated the highest in terms of "dissatisfaction". The Director of Nursing is taking the lead in resolving the issues around discharge.

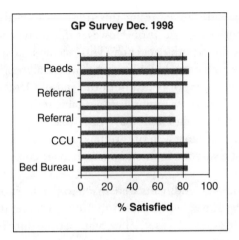

Fig. 11 A sample of the GP Survey Results

As well as corporate feedback, the Divisions have also developed their own mechanisms. For instance, the Cardiothoracic Division has now held 3 focus groups, gaining feedback on their services and have as a consequence devised an information booklet. The feedback has been particularly useful in identifying areas where patients would like more choice, and how much information the patient would like about their operation. Additional learning has been around "how" to organise and run a focus group. The lessons learnt have been presented to the Customer Satisfaction Steering Group, which has representation from every area of the Trust. Similarly, the Division of Women and Children held a series of focus groups, to obtain feedback on the current maternity services and to test women's opinions of future changes in service provision.

2.22.4 Staff surveys

As with the other steering groups, the Staff Satisfaction Steering Group was initially formulated in 1996, following that first corporate assessment. The key aim was to identify staff satisfiers and dissatisfiers factors, and design a staff satisfaction questionnaire to measure the same. The group originally comprised a cross section of staff representing all professions and staff groups. Each member of the Staff Satisfaction Steering Group was responsible for holding focus groups amongst their peers to identify the main satisfiers and disatisfiers for that group of staff. This was distilled and then prioritised into a single list, which was incorporated in the design of the questionnaire.

The first Trust wide survey using this tool was carried out in May 1997, following an initial pilot in April. However the analysis took several months due to the time taken with data entry. This role was carried out by one of the members of the Staff Satisfaction Steering Group, alongside other duties. The Corporate results were not issued until the end of October 1997. Individual Divisional and Directorate results were available in March/April of 1998. The Staff Satisfaction Steering Group have reviewed the process of managing this exercise. The need for a more timely process has been met by the appointment of a survey administrator, to manage corporate surveys.

During the review, amendments were made to the questionnaire, as well as to the process. The survey was repeated in 1999. A better distribution method resulted in a better response rate. The Staff Satisfaction Steering Group have since made recommendations on targets for improvement to the Developing Excellence Steering Group, which in turn have been incorporated in the "Business Planning Assumptions" guidance.

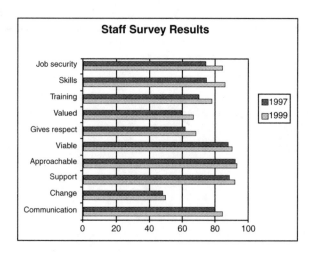

Fig. 12. Sample of Staff Survey Results

As mentioned earlier, there is now a dedicated staff member that deals with the corporate surveys, and a rolling programme is in place to ensure that surveys are carried out at different times of the year. The customer and staff satisfaction steering groups have now combined. They meet every two to three months to oversee and review the survey process.

2.22.5 Key performance results

In respect of the above, it is necessary to point out that a 'Business' Results Steering Group was initially established in 1996. (The EFQM model used the term business results at the time). The group debated what the Key Business Results (now Key Performance Results) for the Trust should be. The group found these difficult to define. This was largely due to the group working separately to the other steering groups and felt unable to define tangible targets, until the other groups had specified their respective processes and targets.

In 1998/9, significant progress was made in clarifying Key Performance Results required at Directorate, Divisional and Corporate levels. This work linked to the national developments for recording and monitoring service results and national standards. As a result of very successful pilots, it was agreed to develop this approach across the Trust for all Directorates and Divisions. This has been a key development for Clinical Governance. The Trust believes the Excellence Model does provide a robust framework for Clinical Governance. The principles that underpin the Excellence Model run parallel with those of Clinical Governance.

A good specific example is that of the Directorate of Obstetrics which has developed an innovative system of critical incident analysis. The process leader, a midwife with a law degree, investigates all complaints, critical incidents, college recommendations, and any other relevant concerns. Any member of staff can refer an issue into the process. The midwife produces a report for discussion. The Clinical Director and the Maternity Services Manager meet fortnightly to discuss issues pending, (usually between 8-10) and if necessary they involve other relevant parties. The midwife has a session on the monthly clinical audit meeting. Recommendations and changes in practice are documented and shared with other members of the Directorate.

Another significant development in 1998/9 was an emphasis on evidence based practice. Clinical teams throughout the Trust have been supported with expert help and the development of team based approach to the critical appraisal of the latest research has commenced. Throughout 2000, the development will continue and will focus on priority areas for the Trust.

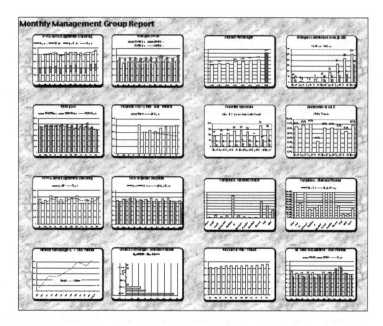

Fig. 13. The Management Group Report – Key Performance Results

At a corporate level, the group has produced a draft set of key performance results to be presented to the management group on a monthly basis. The report displayed in Fig. 13 is two sides of A3. This has replaced copious documents on activity, finance and manpower, which used to form part of the management group report. The new key performance report was introduced in March 2000.

2.23 Integrating Developing Excellence across the Trust and wider afield

The acid test of any framework is on demonstrable results. We now wish to summarise results of the wider application of the Excellence Model, both inside and outside the Trust. In a case study of this kind, it is difficult to deal comprehensively with all results, nor for that matter include all instances of results. At the outset though, one fact is indisputable. All areas of the Trust are actively involved in improvement activity in relation to Developing Excellence. Word limit pressures make it impossible to include all of these and we apologise to colleagues whose area or project has not been included.

2.23.1   Division of Surgery

The Directorate of General Surgery was one of the three pilot areas for the Excellence Model. Using the Excellence Model brought about a number of improvements to both the care of patients and to the working environment for staff. For instance, the refurbishment of the surgical floor at South Cleveland Hospital involving staff in the new design, has created patient and visitor friendly nurse stations.

Recently, the Ophthalmology Directorate within Surgery increased the number of patients having day case cataract surgery. Now 85% of the 1,800 patients that the Directorate treats with cataracts each year, are treated as day cases. Beds have now been replaced with reclining chairs and new methods of carrying out cataract surgery, performed by all the ophthalmologists in the department, means that having a cataract removed is as easy as going to the dentist. This type of surgery, carried out under local anaesthetic pioneered at the Trust's North Riding Infirmary, is ideal for older patients with other medical conditions, which makes general anaesthetic unsuitable.

The Division had an opportunity to alter its structure to reflect process re-design that was carried out. A Specialist Nurse/Process Manager has been appointed in Ophthalmology, ENT, and Urology and acts as the co-ordinator for process reviews currently being undertaken. An extensive training programme and ongoing support has been provided to these personnel. A lead nurse for the whole Division has also been appointed and is leading on an F & G Grade Leadership programme, with support from both Leadership and Organisation Development.

The Division is also using the Excellence Model to redesign its Outpatient Department, in line with the Government and Trust's targets of over 13-week waiters.

The Breast Care Team used the principles of Excellence to improve care for patients with breast disease. They mapped out the processes in the Outpatient Department, developed a team approach with Acute and Community services, devised patient held records and devised a multi-disciplinary pathway of care, with one set of notes for each patient containing all clinical information. The team has successfully implemented the 2 week waiting target for Breast Cancer.

2.23.2   Division of Medicine

Here recognition will be made of outcomes relating to emergency medical admissions. In 1998, 35 consultants working in Medicine and senior nurses from within the speciality, agreed to reconfigure medicine using this approach. Five teams were set up to ensure that emergency admissions received a faster diagnosis from a suitable specialist with more support staff, such as pathology and mental health nurses, in attendance. Skill mix of staff on post acute wards was altered, so that more qualified nurses were available at the acute stage.

As a result of these measures, the average time spent in hospital has fallen by one full day since 1998.

Other successes include :

40% of emergency admissions are discharged in the first 24 hours (10% two years ago);

activity is up by 6% using 4.5% fewer bed days;

readmission's after discharge are down from 7.5% to 6.5%;

sickness absence rates have fallen below the Trust average and currently there are no vacancies.

The Division has appointed a project manager to co-ordinate the Divisions application of the Excellence Model and self assessment.

2.23.3   Division of Cardiothoracic Services

The Division of Cardiothoracic Services has used a process review to analyse the working of the surgical pre-admissions clinic. Pre-admission activities including blood tests are carried out 2-3 days before. The patient attends pre admission assessment with their relatives, to discuss the nature of the surgery and to organise discharge.

An outpatient review in Cardiothoracic Services took place in 1999, to look at the use of clinics and a reduction of Did Not Attends (DNAs). The Division went on to review its existing facilities and systems, and to consider improvements to its services, such as near patient testing.

The Division has its own Developing Excellence Steering Group and has reviewed and developed action plans for a number of topics, including :

- *a Customer Satisfaction working party*
- *patient focus groups*
- *patient suggestion boxes*
- *an Impact on Society link person who has done presentations to colleagues in the Division, on recycling, bicycle usage, etc.*

The Division also has conducted a review of Post Myocardial Infarction stress testing. The stress test aims to identify those at risk of a further ischaemic event. A number of patients were being tested following discharge to prevent bed blocking. However, this caused delays of up to 178 days in the test being carried out in the outpatients department. Reorganisation of the clinics has led to better utilisation of staff and patients' time, thereby increasing the number of tests performed.

2.23.4   Division of Women and Children

- **Colposcopy Clinic**

The medically led Colposcopy Service, with 750 new referrals each year, already exceeded all the national standards. However, staff felt they could do even better if the clinic was more efficient. All the staff involved in the process, led by the consultant plus a local GP, met to review and redesign the process. The process was redesigned based around, what patients wanted for the service; the positive clinical evidence available about the benefits of a 'see and treat' for certain patients; and on what would provide rewarding jobs for staff. The result is a clinically led service supported by a Nurse Colposcopist. Through discussion with all local GPs, a new process of referral and recall for consultation was agreed.

Evaluation of the new processes have demonstrated radical improvement including:

- *direct referral from cytology means that the time taken to generate appointments has reduced from 13.5 days to 24 hours*
- *consultation time increased from 10 minutes to 30 minutes*
- *there is patient choice for 'see and treat' service, with a less than 10% over treatment rate*
- *the waiting times for new referrals is between 2-4 weeks*
- *the DNA rate is down from 20% to 10%*
- *unnecessary smears have reduced by 100%*
- *patient, GP and Staff Satisfaction is very high.*

The significant improvements in patient care provided by the Colposcopy service has been recognised by a Charter Mark award.

- **Obstetrics – A Whole Directorate approach**

Staff working within the Obstetric Directorate have always been willing to examine and change practice. There is a genuine commitment to improve services to patients. The Clinical Director was involved in the early pilots and firmly believed that using the Excellence Model would provide the means of delivering significant changes required in response to the advances in practice, that are both internally and externally driven.

The project aims initially were to

- *Apply the Excellence Model as a means of ensuring, that services are managed in a systematic fashion which ensures delivery of consistently high standards of care to patients, and is based upon the principle of continuous improvement;*
- *Increase organisational understanding of the application of the model in its entirety within a health care environment.*

The commitment made:

The cost of the project implementation was borne by the directorate;
The staff working in Women and Children delivered the project's vision with outside support when necessary;
Current best practice was retained and enhanced and the project was to be conducted in a way that involved all of the staff.

Benefits to date :

For patients –

A more patient focused maternity care
Improved choice, continuity and control
Midwifery-led care for low dependence patients
More opportunities for integrated midwifery care
More focused and better resourced high dependency and critical care.

For staff :

Improved staff satisfaction
A motivated, flexible, highly skilled workforce
Reducing sickness and absence, and recruitment and retention problems
Increased involvement in decision making processes.

For the organisation:

Robust and sustainable processes for all key activities
Clearly defined and monitored performance targets
Improved utilisation and control of resources
Whole directorate working at 'best in class' standard.

2.23.5 Finance Directorate

Staff in the Finance Directorate have mapped their monthly finance processes. They have revised some of these processes, set targets for improvement and have put together recommendations for presentation to their colleagues in the department and for the Regional office.

A group of staff in the Finance Directorate have mapped the flow of A, B and C forms (for new starters, change of circumstances and leavers). They have redesigned the route for the forms as well as redesigning the forms.

The invoice processing system has improved dramatically since the group took a fresh look at it through Developing Excellence. From a base of 44% of invoices paid within 30 days, the Trust now pays 86% of its invoices within 30 days.

There is currently a group looking at the process flow of capital finances in a bid to rationalise timescales and storage of paper based data, in preparation for the move onto a single site. The Directorate use self assessment against the Excellence Model to identify areas for improvement. In the past they have used workshop and proforma approaches. However, they are currently putting together a substantial document of evidence to use for the next assessment.

2.23.6 Division of Neurosciences

The Division is a pilot area for the development of the Nursing Strategy. They have established eight project teams to look at key processes involved in the development of nursing into the 21st century. They are :

- *Career pathways – succession planning and mentoring*
- *Role definition, structures of nursing*
- *Recruitment and retention*
- *Leadership/professionalism*
- *Education and academic research*
- *Communications*
- *Impact of nursing on other professions/scope of practice*
- *Clinical governance.*

In line with the Corporate Leadership Development Programme, the Division is establishing its own leadership development. The Division used the methodology of Developing Excellence to conduct a focused project examining Clinical Governance issues for patients with malignant intracranial glioma and pituitary adenoma. This work has highlighted a number of service improvements that will be addressed. The intention is to disseminate this good practice internally and externally via a regional Beacon Day event. There are also a number of other key outcomes including:

Policy and Strategy – *The division is developing its own policies such as induction, bed utilisation, sickness absence, training and development.*

Process Redesign – *Ongoing work for the delivery of angiography services and neurology outpatients.*

People – *The division is revising staffing structures for the ward areas, i.e. who is needed for what roles and responsibilities, and at what grades. The division has also used Developing Excellence to develop a framework for competency based job descriptions.*

Policy and Strategy and Key Performance Results – *The Division, on behalf of the Trust, developed a business planning pro-forma which will enable the plan to operate as a working document, which can be monitored throughout the year. It also developed a pro-forma business case development form and capital monitoring form.*

2.23.7 Division of Anaesthesia and Theatres

Two parallel process reviews were undertaken within Theatres, concentrating on the patient's journey to and from theatre, and the operating list scheduling process. Following extensive work, which also included patient surveys, a number of results have been achieved:

65% of patients' journeys to and from theatre are now in a chair and not on a trolley. This has led to a major reconstruction of grading with fewer outside Theatre Porters required and no Operating Department Orderlies or Operating Department Assistants. A new integrated Health Care Assistant role has been introduced with core competencies, NVQ's and specialist areas such as recovery and/or scrub.

Three Theatre performance standards are also being introduced :

'Theatre lists will commence on time' - a 25% improvement has been seen in this area.
'Patients will be in the anaesthetic room five minutes prior to list start time' - this has increased from 50% to 70%.
'All areas of patient documentation will be completed as accurately as possible' - this has increased from 37% to 90%.

2.23.8   Division of Trauma

Staff in the Division of Trauma are working on a number of process reviews. They aim to :

- *Improve waiting times and prioritisation for patients needing emergency surgery*
- *Consolidate and improve the various current preoperative and admission processes in the Division*
- *Develop a robust and user-friendly specialty-to-specialty patient referral process*
- *Ensure patients receive good quality up-to-date information at the most appropriate time*
- *Improve and streamline the purchase ordering system specifically focused on ordering prosthesis, ensuring cost benefits are realised.*

The Division has appointed an EFQM Co-ordinator to ensure these projects are realised and to be a resource person to the Division.

2.23.9   Across the Cancer Care Alliance

The Cancer Care Alliance of Teesside, South Durham and North Yorkshire, of which South Tees Acute Hospitals NHS Trust is the Cancer Centre, is using the Excellence Model to improve care and service provision for those with cancer and suspected cancer. A core team works across the Alliance, with the Cancer Units to ensure continuity of service delivery and improvement, and to disseminate good practice between primary, secondary and tertiary care professionals. The Macmillan Service, hospices, GPs, health authorities and social services are also involved.

A Teesside Cancer Collaborative was established in July 2000, utilising Health Action Zone funding, to pump prime the Cancer Modernisation Agenda.

Using the Trust's approach to process re-design, reviews are currently being undertaken within a number of specialities at South Tees. These include lung, colorectal, gynaecology with Head, Neck and Oral cancer and also involve cross boundary working with Darlington Memorial Hospital. A major outcome of the work so far is the 'link nurse' role, which ensures continuity of care, with appropriate support, from referral to discharge.

2.24 What next and beyond

The Trust is moving quickly towards amalgamating all of its services onto one site and into the new building at South Cleveland Hospital. This work already ahead of schedule, will be completed by 2003. Ensuring a smooth transition of staff from the two redundant sites with the minimal disruption to patients, their relatives and the staff, will be critical to the continuous delivery of high quality care. There is also the challenge of increasing number of patients that will need acute hospital care. This puts pressure on our existing capacity, even without this major change. As part of the transition, we will be conducting an organisational review of our infrastructure. This will include the systems and resources required to effectively manage patient flows through elective, emergency, outpatient and day-care patient pathways. Within this review, we will incorporate the work already undertaken in the key support services of Radiology, Pathology and Theatres, where the existing process review and redesign work will be consolidated and linked together.

As a major provider of acute services, our key performance indicators and results achieved will serve as our baseline to ensure that we can continue to improve our performance against national and regional targets. The recent launch of the National Plan has now identified key standards and requirements for the NHS and we will be using the Excellence Model to assess how closely we meet these requirements.

Each Division and Directorate will now be using the Excellence Model as the framework to produce their business plan. The Model will help to ensure that we take a whole systems approach to implementing and managing change, at all levels throughout the organisation.

2.25 Internal and external achievements

Since 1996, STAHT has carried out three corporate self-assessments and delivered a major Organisation Development programme, which is still ongoing. STAHT now uses bi-annual self-assessment, to review its overall approach and deployment. This informs the subsequent development agenda.

In 1999, STAHT was recognised as one of three National Specialist Learning Centres within the NHS. This was primarily because of STAHT use of the Excellence Model as part of its approach to Organisation Development.

Early in 2000, the Trust was approached by the Northern and Yorkshire NHSE, to provide leadership in developing a region-wide Learning Alliance. In order that this additional goal is achieved, the Learning Centre has changed its name to THE NORTHERN AND YORKSHIRE LEARNING ALLIANCE and as such will undertake three main streams of work:

The National Learning Contract (South Tees)
The Northern and Yorkshire Learning and Service Improvement Contract
Consultancy Support.

The Trust is also a Beacon Site for training and development for Clinical Governance. The past six months have been both successful and demanding for the Learning Centre. Through the Learning Centre, STAHT has shared its experiences with up to 300 delegates, through conferences and has provided consultancy and support for 70 NHS organisations.

The Trust has learnt a great deal over the last six years and increasingly, we receive requests for visits or for presentations at national seminars and conferences. The Trust also learns from others within and outside the NHS, as active members of national and local networking groups. With an emphasis on improving results for patients and a sharp awareness of the pressures and realities of strained resources on complex processes, a culture of commitment, involvement and enthusiasm now prevails.

2.26   Benefits, key to success and lessons learnt
The following is a summary of the benefits, keys to success and lessons learnt.

The benefits: The EFQM Excellence Model has enabled us to:

Systematically identify strengths and areas for improvement, based on evidence and not assumptions

Develop a common understanding of what we are trying to achieve

Increase the rate of continuous improvement and opportunities for radical change

Engage staff in driving change forward

Enthuse staff, develop teams and promote continuous learning

Recognise the need for ownership of performance standards

Share good ideas and best practice

Demonstrate real evidence of improvement

Compare ourselves with others

Measure progress

To have a framework for integrating all our development activity and focus our effort and resources.

Keys to Success

Based on our experiences, we can conclude that success requires:

* *Commitment from the Chief Executive from the very beginning*
* *Stability and consistency in the top team*
* *Clear guidelines and strong project management focus for every project*
* *A champion at Trust Board level to have constant visibility*
* *Focus on quality and improvement, rather than the Excellence Model*
* *Involvement of clinicians from the early stages*
* *Resources (the Trust allocated substantial financial resources to the programme)*
* *Recognition that organisation development is very important if the infrastructure is to be right for step improvements*
* *A gradual start. Demonstrate that dramatic improvements to patients and staff can be achieved by this approach. Gain some expertise and credibility before deploying the approach organisation wide.*

Lessons learnt

We have learnt that:

> *The Excellence Model is not a magic wand. It is a tool, a means to an end, not an end in itself.*
> *It is very time consuming especially for clinical staff who have other major demands*
> *Not to call it EFQM or any other name that will be seen as another initiative or management talk*
> *To choose willing departments initially, i.e. those that want to use it and demonstrate results*
> *It is not a quick fix, nor is it dot to dot management. It is a flexible framework of excellence that allows self examination and it can be used in many different ways.*

We believe the application of the EFQM Model in the NHS has the potential to dramatically improve the way we deliver health care.

We began with a view from the top and we will end in the same way.

> *"If this Trust scored 217 points against the Excellence Model criteria in 1995, whilst being considered an effective and efficient health care organisation, just imagine what we will be like when we score 700!"*

Bill Murray OBE, Chief Executive

Reference
* Hammer, M., and Champy, J.1994. Reengineering the Corporation: A Manifesto for Business Revolution. Nicholas Brearley Publishing Ltd.

Case Study 3

Wakefield and Pontefract Community Health NHS Trust

making a difference

3.1 The context

Wakefield and Pontefract Community Health NHS Trust (WPCHT) provides services mainly to the population of Wakefield Metropolitan District in West Yorkshire. Any of the 320,000 local residents are likely to use our services at some time during their lives. We provide a range of inpatient, outpatient and community based services including:

- Mental Health Services (specialising in care of children and adolescents, people of a working age and older people)
- Learning Disability Services
- Primary Care and Specialist Services, including District Nursing, Health Visiting, Podiatry (Chiropody), Dentistry, Speech and Language Therapy, Community Medical Services, Dietetics, Community Paediatrics, Wheelchair Services
- Forensic Medium Secure Services – The Yorkshire Centre for Forensic Psychiatry specialises in the assessment and treatment of mentally disordered offenders from the whole of the Yorkshire region.

We provide these services from over 50 different sites, including hospitals, clinics and health centres. We also provide services in schools, GP practices, residential homes and people's own homes. To deliver this diverse range of services, the Trust employs approximately 2000 staff, including doctors, nurses, therapists, psychologists, administrative staff and non-clinical support staff.

Since its inception, the Trust has witnessed significant changes in its local environment. In particular, the changes include General Practitioners within Primary Care Groups having a wider role to influence decisions about which services they commission and provide. Initially exercised through the fundholding scheme (100% of the district's general practices were fundholders – the highest take up in the country at the time), GP influence is now vested in Primary Care Groups and, from 2001, Primary Care Trusts. Also, the government drive towards giving GPs a stronger role in planning and delivering NHS services means community nursing staff, who already work as part of GP practice teams, are likely to have to take on broader responsibilities in response to the requirements of GPs.

From the outset, the Trust has recognised the importance of having a clear understanding of its customers, their requirements, and the vagaries of the market, and has demonstrated its commitment to continuous quality improvement in a number of ways. Key quality improvement milestones in the early years can be seen in the table below:

Our Quality Journey: 1993 - 1995

Trust formed	April 1993
Quality Strategy agreed by Trust Board	September 1993
Quality Council formed	September 1993
Audit, research, CQI agendas established	October 1993
CQI training for all staff initiated	November 1993
'Quality Tapestry' handbook produced	November 1993
Communication Strategy implemented	January 1994
Celebration of Quality established (e.g. awards, exhibition)	October 1994
Local Patient's Charter developed	October 1994
Investors in People status achieved	March 1995
Quality, Evaluation & Development (QED) department formed	April 1995
Quality models/frameworks reviewed	July 1995
Charter Mark achieved	December 1995

3.2   Choosing the Model

The review of quality improvement models and frameworks that began in the summer of 1995 sought to bring a sense of cohesion and integration to the Trust's approach to continuous improvement. After an initial consideration of ISO 9000, models based more on the principles of TQM (Total Quality Management) held more appeal, since they reflected a more holistic view of organisations and reflected our existing philosophy and achievements. The Malcolm Baldrige National Award Criteria framework - the most widely used framework in the world at the time - was a serious contender. However, the more recently developed Business Excellence Model (as it was then commonly known), developed by the European Foundation for Quality Management, was the first total quality based self-assessment framework to place an emphasis on business results. In July 1995, a British Quality Foundation accredited consultant gave a presentation to the Trust's Corporate Management Team on the potential strategic benefits of using the Model as a business-planning tool. Following this, the Trust decided to adopt the Business Excellence Model as a self-assessment framework, and later that year, the Trust's first self-assessment team was established.

3.3 Self-assessment

In common with many organisations, a primary reason for adopting the Excellence Model was to use it as a framework for self-assessment. The self-assessment process, as defined by the EFQM in its promotional literature, is:

> '...a comprehensive, systematic and regular review of an organisation's activities and results against a model of excellence. Self-assessment allows the organisation to discern clearly its strengths as well as areas in which improvements can be made and culminates in planned improvement actions, which are then monitored for progress.'

Self-assessment promised many things. The British Quality Foundation's Guide to the Excellence Model (1995), for instance, suggested that the benefits might include:

- a rigorous and structured approach to continuous improvement
- an assessment based on facts and not individual perception
- a means to educate people in the organisation on how to apply the principles of business excellence
- a means to integrate the various quality initiatives into normal business operations
- a powerful diagnostic tool
- an objective assessment against a set of excellence criteria which has become widely accepted across Europe
- a means of measuring progress over time through periodic self assessment
- process-induced improvement activity focused on what is most needed
- a methodology for all levels, from individual business units up to the organisation as a whole
- opportunities to promote and share excellent approaches between different areas of the organisation or, on a wider scale, with other organisations of a similar or diverse nature
- a link between what the organisation needs to achieve and how it puts in place strategies and processes to deliver its objectives
- a means to benchmark internally and externally.

By taking this approach, therefore, we were able to both build on the work undertaken and successes achieved so far, and take a more focused approach to assessing our achievements and action planning for improvement.

3.3.1 Self-assessment - the first time

Typically, self-assessment involves a number of key stages, all of which need to be addressed before proceeding to the next stage, and our own approach followed this sequence. These stages are shown below:

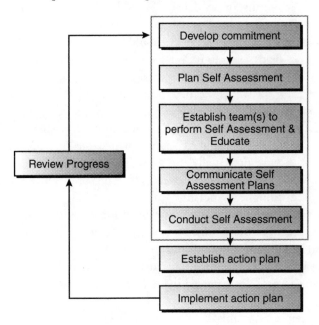

Source: EFQM

Fig. 1 The self-assessment process

3.3.2 Commitment

Within the Trust, the commitment to self-assessment against the Excellence Model from the Chief Executive and members of his Corporate Management Team was strong and explicit. As described above, the decision to adopt the model was based on thorough groundwork, and a wide understanding of the organisation and its readiness to adopt its framework. The importance of having such commitment from the start cannot be overemphasised.

3.3.3 Planning - what approach to take?

Intending to realise many of the proposed benefits described earlier, the Trust needed to decide, from a host of possibilities, the approach it should take to carrying out its first self-assessment. Should the self-assessment be based on a questionnaire to be completed by identified staff (being quick to administer and analyse, and without the need to score); should it be a perception-based workshop (requiring little advanced preparation on the part of the participants); or should it take the form of an 'award-simulation', based on the painstaking gathering of 'evidence'? Should self-assessment initially be tried out at a departmental level, to determine the viability of carrying out a corporate-wide exercise? How detailed should the self-assessment be? How much time should be devoted to it? Who should be actively involved in it?

The answer to these questions was determined in large part by the objectives the self-assessment was hoping to achieve, and the preferred approach of the Corporate Management Team. A major rationale for adopting the model at the time was as a management tool. Consequently, the first self-assessment exercise needed to have potentially the most impact in identifying how the organisation could be managed more effectively. The approach also needed to recognise that although 'ownership' of the process by the Corporate Management Team was essential, their workloads made it unfeasible for any of them to be members of the self-assessment team. It was also recognised that the assessment might best be carried out by a group of people with less of a vested interest in achieving a 'strongly positive' outcome. In January 1996, the Corporate Management Team agreed the following objectives:

- To carry out an organisation-wide self-assessment, establishing an assessment baseline
- To identify organisational strengths and areas for improvement, and to present feedback on these to the Corporate Management Team
- To feed improvement opportunities into the business planning cycle, including corporate objectives
- To provide data to share with benchmarking partners
- To develop the process of self-assessment using the Excellence Model as an annual part of the business planning process.

In conjunction with the identified members of the self-assessment team, an action plan was agreed to enable the above objectives to be achieved. The action plan detailed how the required evidence on which to assess the organisation's strengths and areas for improvement would be obtained, drawing on a range of information sources:

- Paper sources, e.g. policies, plans, strategies, quality improvement project reports, feedback reports. Trust Board papers were seen to be a particularly rich source of evidence, providing, for example:

  Quarterly Reports - HR Reports showing equal opportunities information, sickness absence rates, productivity; Quality Monitoring Reports showing trend information against National and Local Charter Standards, and Health Authority Contracting Standards; Business Plan Monitoring Reports showing achievement against Business Plan Objectives and Complaints Monitoring Reports.

  Monthly Reports - on Performance Management; Contract Monitoring (Finance & Activity) and Finance Monitoring;
  Ad Hoc Reports - Capital Expenditure Against Capital Programmes; Site Utilisation Study and Media Reports.

- Interviews with the Chief Executive and Directors
- Focus groups with staff representing a range of services/professional backgrounds
- Award submissions (e.g. Investors in People, Charter Mark, National Training Awards).

3.3.4   Establishing the self-assessment team

In the process of planning for the event, six individuals were subsequently trained, by a BQF-accredited assessor trainer, to form the Trust's self-assessment team. The members of the team were selected on the basis of a number of criteria: all reported to an Executive Director and collectively gave a representative coverage of the Trust's directorates; all were considered to have the necessary knowledge, skills and organisational understanding to work productively as a team; all were well able to challenge, to question, to argue their case in presenting evidence, and to change their views in the light of disconfirming evidence presented to them. They were also interested in doing the job from a developmental point of view.

An Executive Director also underwent the training. It was considered desirable that a Director having a more detailed understanding of the Model should act as an important link between the self-assessment team and the Corporate Management Team throughout the duration of the exercise, and subsequently to help the Corporate Management Team interpret key issues in the context of the model. This Director also chaired review meetings following each self-assessment. These meetings evaluated the effectiveness of the self-assessment process and, where indicated, proposed refinements to it.

3.3.5 Communicating the plans

A vexed question here is that of who needed to know that self-assessment was about to be launched on an unsuspecting organisation? Was it necessary to inform the whole organisation? Did people really want to know about it? The organisation had recently been involved (albeit successfully) in a number of initiatives, such as Investors in People and Charter Mark, (perceived initiative-overload threatened), and self-assessment was seen very much as a management tool. The decision was taken, therefore, to keep the process itself relatively low key. That is, there would be no 'big bang' launch of the Excellence Model into the organisation.

What was necessary to be communicated though, was the likely impact that the diversion of time and energies of the self-assessment team would have on its members' normal operational roles. This is important. None of us had the luxury of taking regular blocks of 'time-out' from our everyday jobs to work on the self-assessment. We had to be aware, therefore, that work might need to be re-prioritised. Time had to be protected to gather and review the evidence. Some other work might need to be delegated, and some deadlines might have to be negotiated. In the final stages of the self-assessment process in particular, accessibility to team members - from their subordinates, their peers, their managers - might be curtailed significantly, and people's expectations might need to be managed accordingly.

The self-assessment plans also needed to be communicated to those people across the organisation on whom we would rely to provide us with, or give access to, any sources of evidence which we needed to carry out the self-assessment effectively. An explicit understanding at the start of the process was that we should have unrestricted access to any information we considered relevant, on the basis that confidentiality would be protected and that we would use our professional integrity, in deciding how to deal with any sensitive material. What we did not want, given that time was a valuable resource that none of us could afford to waste, was to encounter barriers in trying to access information. The line management structure - often starting at Director level, was often the main route used to pave the way for the self-assessment team to request any necessary information. In an organisation of around 2000 staff, and with members of the self-assessment team known to be part of one directorate seeking information from another, this preparation was crucial.

Other than communicating the self-assessment plans to those referred to above, the rest of the organisation was largely unaware that the exercise was due to begin. This was considered appropriate at the time. As the use of the model became much more embedded in the organisation though, and its versatility enabled it to be used for purposes other than self-assessment (see later sections), communications about it became commensurately wider, deeper and more detailed.

3.3.6   Conducting the self-assessment

The action plan referred to above detailed roles, responsibilities and timescales. It included, for example, who would be responsible for setting up the interviews and focus groups, who would facilitate and who would take notes, and how the combined information would be shared with other members of the team. A co-ordinator was nominated within the group to ensure that the action plan kept on track, arranged regular review meetings, and kept the link Director updated on progress. A 'resource room' was appropriated, to house the collection of documentary evidence that had been identified and collected. All the documentation was reviewed by each member of the self-assessment team. Supplemented by the findings of the interviews and focus groups, the documentary evidence was assessed individually by each member of the team, who then allocated a score against each of the criterion parts based on the nature of this collective evidence. The process was challenging and taxing, and was spread over several weeks.

3.3.7   Consensus

Having individually scored the organisation against the Model's criteria, based on the gathered evidence, the self-assessment team took themselves off-site for two days for a 'consensus meeting'. This is where teamwork abilities come into their own! Scoring is, of course, not an exact science, and individuals can allocate very different scores based on what seems like the same evidence. People interpret facts differently, have different concepts of 'excellence', are more predisposed than others to score generously, to give the benefit of the doubt etc. An individual's position within the organisation can influence markedly how they see 'deployment'. Professional interests and roles may lead some to become defensive in certain areas. Some will have expert knowledge on some topics, but have very limited awareness of how things are actually done, as opposed to how things should be, on areas beyond their day-to-day remit.

Personalities inevitably come into it as well. A forceful individual may exert influence over other team members based on their talents of persuasion, rather than on the weight of evidence. And evidence is the key - the whole purpose of the consensus meeting is to come to an agreement on what the evidence is saying, and not on anecdote, wishful thinking, or self-interest.

Despite such potential obstacles, the two-day event was a constructive and stimulating exercise. That isn't to say there was no disagreement - in fact, debate became quite heated at times. But at the end of the session, all team members were happy that the identified list of strengths, areas for improvement, and score, gave a fair and realistic 'snapshot' of where the organisation was at that particular time, referenced against the Excellence Model.

3.3.8 Feedback and establishing the action plan

An important precursor to developing an action plan was to feed back the findings of the self-assessment to the Corporate Management Team, in such a way that they accepted the legitimacy of them. A presentation to the Corporate Management Team by the self-assessment team was made in June 1996, accompanied by a written report. This was a meeting that required thoughtful preparation! The credibility of the assessment team was at stake, as was the acceptability of the Excellence Model as a management tool in the eyes of the Directors.

The self-assessment was the most thorough, searching and testing organisational diagnosis that had been carried out. Evidence of good practice was identified, captured in the report, and needed to be recognised and built upon. Inevitably though, the exercise revealed many areas where there was scope for improvement. For example, under 'Processes', the feedback report stated that:

There is no evidence of systematic identification of critical processes, or definition, or design. There is no process for identifying processes. There is no explicit understanding of processes, and no explicit review of them.

An area for improvement in the 'People Satisfaction' section of the report stated that:

There is no evidence of the organisation systematically assessing its people's satisfaction. All evidence is anecdotal. There is consequently no data to monitor the satisfaction of our staff over time, and therefore no trends can be discerned.

The reference point for how the feedback was reported and presented was the scoring guidance of the Model. That is, that high scores cannot be given for evidence that is at best anecdotal, irrespective of 'gut feeling' or how much we 'know to be true'. This was a bitter pill for some to swallow. Once the presentation had been made, the self-assessment team worked with the Corporate Management Team at identifying priorities for improvement.

3.3.9　Implementing the action plan

It was originally intended that the areas targeted in drawing up the action plan should have been incorporated into the Directors' objectives, and into the Business Plan. The misalignment between the timing of the self-assessment process and the Business Planning cycle, though, meant that some targeted improvement areas did not receive the level of attention that they otherwise might have done, resulting in some attrition in impact. However, some important and enduring actions were taken, in the light of the agreed importance of the identified 'gaps' revealed by the self-assessment.

Example 1 - Processes
All the Directors worked with members of the assessment team during the following year in identifying key processes and associated sub-processes. The following high-level action plan was used to aid the development of this work:

• Corporate key process and sub-process map signed off by Corporate Management Team including Directors' personal responsibility for key processes

- Implementation of a programme of work to facilitate process improvements, including:
  - -training of other staff
  - -identification of local process 'champions' to help promote and embed the approach into the Trust culture and to pilot the approach
  - -use of appropriate training opportunities for process improvement, for example, for service clinicians who receive training in the development of 'care pathways'
- Monitoring and review using self-assessment against the Excellence Model.

The fishbone diagram below describes the outcome of this early work, which formed the basis of continued focus on process management and process improvement, following a major deficit in this area identified by our first self-assessment.

Fig. 2 Key and sub-process diagram

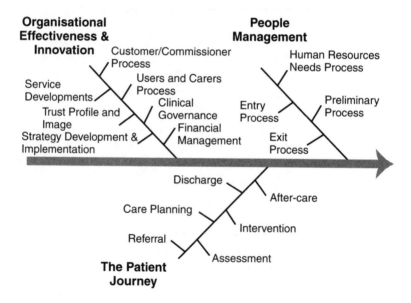

Example 2 - Staff Opinion Survey
Following the first self-assessment, and the identified gap in evidence of perception data from staff, a staff opinion survey was designed and piloted. A

disappointingly low response rate (24%) to the first survey led to improvements in the approach taken to both disseminate, and promote the importance of the survey. A 43% response rate to the survey in the second year was followed by response rates at around 50% for the most recent surveys. (In the spirit of the Model, the survey is reviewed annually, targets have been set, and trend data is now collected and used to drive improvements).

3.3.10 Reviewing Progress

The final stage in the self-assessment steps described earlier in the chapter is the review of progress, based on the action plans that stemmed from the identified strengths and areas for improvement. Whilst a review process was built into all the improvement initiatives to come out of the first self-assessment, a review of the overall self-assessment process was conducted in advance of preparing for the next.

3.4 Learning Points - The second self-assessment and beyond

• The Excellence Model and its relevance to health care

In reviewing how much the first self-assessment had lived up to our expectations, and whether or not the intention to make self-assessment an annual event still made sense, we needed to reflect on the Model's relevance to us. We knew that the model's private sector origins had proved to be an obstacle to some public sector organisations generally. Indeed, there was evidence that the 'business speak' that sprinkled parts of the original Model had served to put off some organisations in other sectors from adopting it, in its current form at the time. Our own experience was that the Model was entirely suitable when applied to a health care setting. There were occasions when the meaning behind some of the language needed to be interpreted slightly differently, but this was by no means a major issue. All the indications were that self-assessment using the Model was as effective, robust, and systematic as the promotional material had claimed. (The revised, 1999, Model has changed some of the language to address initial concerns about its transferability to public/not-for-profit organisations.)

• Time, energy and commitment

What we almost certainly under-estimated as new recruits to the self-assessment process was how much time and energy the whole exercise would demand. Subsequent self-assessments have attempted to make the process more efficient - e.g. through more selectivity in what information is collected, by allocating tasks more widely and more equitably, by planning ahead more effectively and protecting time better, and generally being more focused.

What also has become increasingly evident is how much commitment is needed to sustain the process. Principally, the active and explicit commitment of the Chief Executive was fundamental to continuing with self-assessment long enough for it to demonstrate benefits and for it to become embedded into the organisation. Given all the other things competing for attention, without that commitment there is little doubt that adopting the Excellence Model for self-assessment would have been consigned to the failed initiatives scrap heap. The commitment needs to go much wider, though. Certainly, there needs to be commitment from all members of the assessment team, otherwise the whole process would just become a chore, and some members of the team would end up carrying an unfair burden of the workload. There also needs to be commitment from all those who have an input into the self-assessment process, at whatever level within the organisation. Constantly having to chase people up who have not provided promised information for an assessor is not rewarding, and causes avoidable frustration and pressure. Finally, the line managers of those involved in self-assessment need to be committed to the process, to be able to appropriately support and accommodate the needs of their staff who are engaged in a difficult balancing act.

- **The feedback report - bite but don't bullet**
Our first feedback report was intended to put the relevant information across in an economical way - that is, many of the strengths (in particular) and areas for improvement were one or two word 'bullets'. The assumption was that we all knew what we meant, and so would anybody else who read the report. This is not the case. Also, when it comes to re-visiting the report some months down the line, what seemed like an obvious strength at that time is less obvious as memories struggle to capture the original rationale. The question *'why did we say that last year?'* was not uncommon after the first self-assessment. Subsequent feedback reports have, therefore, been written more fully to explain why an approach/result was seen as a strength. Areas for improvement also needed to be explicit enough to indicate what action might be warranted. This does add time to writing up the report of course, but our experience is that this is time well spent.

- **The tyranny of scoring**

We probably made a tactical error in revealing the first self-assessment scores too early on in the process of feeding back to the Corporate Management Team. Rather than concentrating on the strengths, areas for improvement, and priorities for action, and seeing the scoring mechanism as a guide that brings added rigour into the self-assessment, some people became distracted by the scores. Debate would sometimes then focus on the relative scores, as opposed to the issues themselves. Scoring is too imprecise for it to be the focus of that much attention, in the overall scheme of things. Subsequent self-assessments have relegated revealing the score to later in the feedback process, as an indicator of progress, as a crude 'temperature check', and nothing more sophisticated than that.

- **Champions and cynics**

It would be unrealistic to assume that everyone will embrace a new initiative with equal verve, particularly when so many 'fads' come and go. What was important for us though, during the early days in particular, was to have people in positions of influence, at Director level downwards, willing to champion the cause whilst it got off the ground. What wins the cynics over (and it would be a very unusual organisation that didn't have their share), is not so much trying to persuasively articulate the merits of a particular approach, but through the ability of that approach to demonstrate visible benefits to them. The capacity of the Model to do just that has unfolded with our wider experience of using it.

- **Self-assessment and business planning**

Momentum was lost in several targeted improvement areas following the first self-assessment, because the outcome did not feed into the Business Planning cycle. The timing of subsequent self-assessments has been changed to ensure that it is now linked to the action planning and performance-monitoring framework provided by the Business Planning process. The clear integration between self-assessment outcome and Business Planning process has been a key development, and from our perspective, needs to happen sooner rather than later.

- **The self-assessment team**

The approach that the organisation has chosen to adopt demands a great deal from the self-assessment team. As a minimum, the team has had to be constituted of people who at least get on with each other. Personality clashes, mind games, ego trips, free loading, responsibility shirking, humourless consensus meetings just won't do. Neither will it do to have team members who recoil from challenge - either challenging their peers, or their seniors. Though self-assessment is a challenging, sometimes painful undertaking, the rewards in terms of development and enhanced knowledge are immense, given the right mix of team members. It would be easy to give only a passing thought to team membership, but it warrants the highest consideration. For our part, being members of the self-assessment team itself has tended to be a team-building exercise, and taking part in the annual event has undoubtedly been a taxing yet enjoyable learning opportunity, that has provided a unique insight into the organisation.

In the years following the introduction of the Model into the Trust, the membership of the self-assessment team has changed - there are now more members drawn from clinical backgrounds. New challenges in the 'environment' have also presented themselves, and the Model has been put to the test in its ability to help us meet them. As will be seen later, such is the flexibility of the Model that it is now used in many ways in addition to self-assessment. The clinical expertise now within the self-assessment team, coupled with the discipline provided by the Model, has generated one very fruitful exploration of how the Model can be put to further use. That is, in helping us meet the demands of a particularly searching agenda - clinical governance.

3.5   A new challenge - Clinical Governance

Having learnt from the experience of corporate-level self-assessments, and having recognised the versatility of the Model, we have undertaken a substantial piece of work in using the Model to support the *Clinical Governance* agenda. The introduction of clinical governance into the NHS in the late 1990's brought new challenges to the organisation, along with an opportunity for us to explore further applications of the Excellence Model. Clinical governance brought a renewed NHS focus on local responsibility for clinical quality, set in the context of national standards of service and a national approach to monitoring performance. Clinical governance is defined as:

"A framework through which NHS organisations are accountable for continuously improving the quality of their services, and safeguarding high standards of care by creating an environment in which excellence in clinical care can flourish." ("A First Class Service", 1998)

The document "Clinical Governance: Quality in the new NHS" (Department of Health, 1999), sets clinical governance at the heart of the wider quality and modernisation agenda for the NHS. There was a recognisable use of language and concepts which have clear origins in TQM, which fit well within our existing values and principles and which mirrored our existing approaches to self-assessment:

"...a systematic approach to quality assurance and improvement within a health organisation..." ("Clinical Governance: Quality in the new NHS" 1999)

The main components of clinical governance in relation to NHS Trusts are summarised below:

3.5.1   The main components of Clinical Governance

1. Clear lines of responsibility and accountability for the overall quality of clinical care
2. A comprehensive programme of quality improvement activities
3. Clear policies aimed at managing risks
4. Procedures for all professional groups to identify and remedy poor performance

Source: 'Clinical Governance: Quality in the new NHS', Department of Health, 1999.

The advent of clinical governance meant that for the first time, NHS Trusts would be *held accountable* for quality. Clinical governance is underpinned by a statutory duty requiring NHS Trusts to put and keep in place, arrangements for monitoring and improving the quality of the health care they provide. The focus is on delivering consistently better outcomes for patients – learning from experience, continuously improving the quality of services through systematic approaches. This is as much about culture as it is about systems and process – a focus on developing an organisational culture in which clinical excellence and quality of service are paramount, in an environment of openness and honesty, collaboration and creativity.

As an organisation, it was believed that Clinical Governance provided a natural 'next step' in our quality journey – an opportunity to build on existing structures and processes and to strengthen our continuously developing 'quality culture', through increased accountability and a stronger focus on clinical involvement.

The first stage of the introduction of Clinical Governance involved NHS Trusts establishing leadership, accountability, reporting and working arrangements and formulating a development plan on the basis of a 'baseline assessment' of capabilities and capacities.

As work to understand the impact of Clinical Governance began, it became clear that the Trust's approach to ensuring the systematic delivery of all actions and processes required to support Clinical Governance should naturally be centralised around the Clinical Management Teams (CMTs). There are 10 CMTs within the organisation, each covering a different clinical service area, (e.g. Forensic Services; Child and Adolescent Services; Primary Care Nursing Services). The teams comprise managers and clinicians and have a co-ordination and leadership function for the relevant clinical services. Within this remit, CMTs are responsible for co-ordination of quality planning across their service areas. Therefore, it was argued that CMTs were best placed to understand the service requirements and capabilities and lead the clinical governance baseline assessment process. The baseline assessment was also perceived as an opportunity for the Trust's Clinical Management Teams to take a more central role within the Trust's broader EFQM self-assessment processes and thus have a more direct input to the annual business planning process. This gave us an opportunity to add value to our approach to self-assessment by achieving greater involvement of services. In effect, this new devolved approach to self-assessment could be piloted as part of the Trust's baseline audit exercise.

3.6   Why the Excellence Model?

The suitability of the Model to underpin an assessment of clinical governance was supported by the results of an internal study, carried out for an MA dissertation, which investigated the benefits brought to the organisation of applying the self-assessment process at the level of a single clinical service. This work, carried out by one of the Trust's EFQM assessors, within Specialist Services, concluded that the use of a common approach to assessing the quality of clinical services within the organisation would improve consistency and facilitate co-ordination of the range of existing approaches applied across the services studied. It was also believed that an initiative that continued to recognise the work already done and which was aligned with corporate processes would retain the confidence and commitment of staff.

The approach taken in this study involved the completion of a series of proformas designed to facilitate the gathering of evidence about current performance against the nine criteria of the Model. A simple rating scale was employed to facilitate 'scoring' of performance. Whilst it is acknowledged that there are limitations inherent in the use of scoring tools, the intention was that the mechanism should at least enable identification of strengths and areas for improvement and enable year on year comparisons of performance to be made. The proformas and rating scale were adapted from an approach described by Hakes and Reed (1997), simplified to meet the following criteria:

❖   The assessment tool would have to be suitable for use by clinical leads who do not have detailed knowledge of the Model
❖   The tool should not be overly time-consuming to apply, but would have to demonstrate comprehensive coverage of aspects of service quality
❖   The tool would have to clearly identify strengths and areas for improvement in order to facilitate action-planning.

The study resulted in the development of a simple tool that met the above criteria and enabled a comprehensive assessment of quality within a single clinical service. Subsequent discussions about the need to develop an effective Clinical Governance baseline assessment tool, recognised that there would be many benefits to be had from continuing to use the Model's framework and for using a proforma approach by:

❖ Continuing the Trust experience of self-assessment and benefiting from the expertise of the Trust's self-assessment team in the development and implementation phases
❖ Ensuring alignment with the corporate approach at achieving consistency
❖ Use of a framework that was proven to demonstrate progress over time
❖ Use of a rigorous and structured approach that had already demonstrated organisational benefits
❖ Use of an approach that would enable comprehensive coverage of existing quality initiatives
❖ Developing a format which would support team assessment.

3.7 The baseline assessment tool

A project to develop a clinical governance baseline assessment tool was established. The scope of the project was to identify and implement a process whereby the CMTs could complete the required baseline assessment. A project board and project team comprising senior clinicians, members of the Trust Excellence Model self-assessment team and clinical governance leads were established and the following objectives were identified:

❖ To produce an appropriate assessment tool based on the Excellence Model to be used by the CMTs
❖ To determine and implement an effective process of briefing, training and supporting CMTs to carry out the baseline assessment and produce relevant action plans
❖ To evaluate key stakeholder perceptions of the efficacy of both the audit tool and the training & support process.

There were obvious difficulties for CMTs in undertaking such a key role in the organisational baseline assessment. These difficulties related to the varied levels of operational functioning of individual CMTs and the time constraints on individual CMT members to carry out the task without adverse impact on their clinical commitments. However, the benefits associated with the project were perceived to be far greater than just enabling compliance with the requirement to complete a baseline assessment. It was believed that the work undertaken would assist in the developmental process by which the CMTs would understand and be enabled to deliver on their clinical governance responsibilities. It was seen as an opportunity to facilitate consistency of approach across the ten teams, and to support team-working. It was recognised that the baseline assessment process could enhance the Trust's business planning processes through providing a mechanism for greater service involvement. It was also intended that the use of the assessment tool and development of action plans based on this should underpin the annual quality planning process undertaken by the CMTs.

3.7.1 Assessment tool development - process

There were five stages within the development process:

Stage 1: Identification of the primary CMT functions & responsibilities within clinical governance. (This work was completed in collaboration with the Trust's Director of Corporate Development, who is also the lead Director for Clinical Governance).

Stage 2: Identification and collation of relevant Model's information. (This work was completed in collaboration with qualified Model's assessors within the Trust).

Stage 3: Identification and collation of relevant clinical governance information. (This work was completed with reference to both national and local clinical governance literature).

Stage 4: Identification of key elements to be incorporated within the assessment tool and production of a draft version. (This consisted of a consultative process involving all members of the project team, the lead Director for Clinical Governance, and other key Trust personnel with identified leading roles in relation to clinical governance).

Stage 5: Pilot phase – the assessment tool was reviewed by one CMT and the feedback used to refine the tool before full implementation.

The project team set out to design an assessment tool that would be comprehensive yet uncomplicated and which would meet the requirements of received clinical governance guidance. Given the relatively limited amount of time available to the CMTs to carry out their assessment, it was recognised that a simple scoring mechanism based around a rating scale approach would be most practical. It must be noted however, that the whole process was also seen as a means to pilot the tool with the expectation that changes indicated by the pilot evaluation might well include the development/use of rating scales that would offer greater definition.

The resulting assessment tool consists of two main sections - enablers and results, and a different process of assessment is applied to each.

For each enabler, relevant criteria are given (supported by written guidelines to ensure consistent interpretation) against which the CMTs identified current practice. Excerpts from the 'policy & strategy' section are provided as an example below:

3.7.2 Excerpt from 'Policy and Strategy' and guidelines for completion

2. POLICY & STRATEGY				Guidelines
CRITERIA For all <u>inappropriate criteria</u> write *Not Appropriate'* across the 3 answer boxes. For all criteria you are <u>unable to assess</u> write *'Cannot Answer'* across all 3 answer boxes.	**Tick Relevant box**			1.a. Are all clinical service areas fully covered within the strategy? Does the CMT strategy relate directly to the Trust Values and Principles and the strategic direction given by the Business Plan? Are the Business Plan and relevant Corporate Strategy Documents (e.g. Clinical Effectiveness Strategy, IM&T Strategy) used to help define the CMT strategy?
1. CMT CQI/Quality Strategy Development integrated with the Organisational CQI and Business Planning Programme:	YES	IN PART	NO	
a. The CMT has a clear vision/ strategy for all the clinical service areas covered.				
b. The CMT and clinical service areas have an annual quality/ business plan which identifies their priorities and objectives for the year				1.b. Are the priorities/ objectives clearly stated?

Source: WPCHT Clinical Governance baseline assessment tool, 1999

The CMTs were then required to identify an overall level of achievement in relation to all the given criteria within each enabler, using the rating table shown below:

Rating table for Enabler criteria

	Level 1	Level 2	Level 3	Level 4	Level 5
Planning	Doing Nothing	Just Starting	Systematic planning approach for some criteria	Systematic planning for many criteria	Fully integrated planning for all criteria – normal CMT working practice
Implementation	Not stated	Just starting	Some criteria implemented	Many criteria implemented	All criteria implemented
Evaluation	Non-Existent	Just Starting	Evidence of review and refinement of a few criteria	Regular reviews for most criteria and evidence of some change based on the reviews	All criteria regularly reviewed with clear evidence of changes having been implemented

Source: WPCHT Clinical Governance baseline assessment tool 1999

Finally, the CMTs were required to identify perceived strengths and perceived areas for improvement within each enabler. This formed the basis for the CMTs' action plans. Strengths/areas for improvement might relate to specific criteria such as "the CMT has a clear strategy". However, strengths/areas for improvement might also relate to a particular function e.g., a CMT might feel its strengths lie in planning and implementation, but perceive a need to develop/improve evaluation processes.

The results section required CMTs to identify actual results achieved rather than the approach taken. For each result area, criteria were identified against which the CMTs:

❖ Identified appropriate measures:
- Corporate measures (these were pre-determined for CMTs within the assessment tool), applicable to all services across the Trust, e.g., the Local Patient Charter Survey
- CMT defined measures applicable to all clinical service areas covered by the CMT
- CMT defined measures which are applicable to specific clinical service areas covered by the CMT

CMTs were asked to identify both direct or indirect measures. For example, for patient satisfaction, a direct measure might be the results of a patient survey, whilst an indirect measure might be an analysis of waiting times (i.e., it is predicted that as waiting times grow, patients become less satisfied).

❖ Specified:

- The review period (how frequently a particular measure is used) – 6-monthly, annually, etc.
- Whether Organisational and/or CMT targets (or standards) had been achieved for each measure.
- Whether any results trend had been identified against this measure, plus a brief indication of whether the trend was negative or positive.
- Whether any comparison had been made of the results against other similar providers elsewhere (benchmarking).

❖ Identified an appropriate overall level for that result criterion using the rating table given below.

❖ Indicated any perceived strengths or areas for improvement to provide the basis for action planning.

Rating table for results criteria

	Level 1	Level 2	Level 3	Level 4	Level 5
Measurement	No relevant measures identified	Very few relevant measures identified	Some relevant measures identified and a few audit processes implemented	Several relevant measures identified with audit processes implemented for most of these	Regular audit carried out for a comprehensive set of relevant measures
Trends of Results	Overall negative trends and/or mostly unsatisfactory audit results against organisational and/or/CMT targets/standards.	Some positive trends and/or satisfactory audit results against organisational and/or CMT targets/ standards.	Positive trends over 3+ years and mostly favourable audit results against organisational and/or CMT targets/standards.	Strongly positive trends over 3+ years and mostly favourable audit results against organisational and/or CMT targets/standards.	Strongly positive trends for 5+ years and all audit results excellent against organisational and/or CMT targets/standards.
External Comparisons	No external comparisons made and/or unfavourable comparisons against other organisations.	Favourable comparisons achieved against other organisations for one or two audit results.	Favourable comparisons achieved against external organisations for some audit results.	Favourable comparisons achieved against external organisations for most audit results.	Excellent comparisons with competitors and/or best in class organisations for all audit results.
Evaluation	No evaluation undertaken, OR No indication that the audit programme led to action which had any positive impact on patient health care.	Evaluation indicates the audit programme led to action which had a slight positive impact on patient health care.	Evaluation indicates the audit programme led to action which had some positive impact on patient health care.	Evaluation indicates the audit programme led to changes being implemented which had a significant positive impact on patient health care.	Evaluation indicates the audit programme led to changes being implemented which had a substantial positive impact on patient health care.

Source: WPCHT Clinical Governance baseline assessment tool 1999

3.7.3 Implementation

It was recognised that the CMTs would need considerable help to carry out their assessment. A half day training programme was organised (offered on three different dates in June and July 1999, to facilitate attendance by clinicians) for CMT members. The training consisted of:

- Background & purpose of the baseline assessment
- Description and demonstration of the assessment tool
- Identification of the broader relationship between the CMTs' clinical governance responsibilities and the strategic & business planning processes within the Trust.

Half of the training session time was a facilitated workshop to allow participants the opportunity to consider the practical considerations related to carrying out the assessment. Each CMT identified the key processes the team would have to employ to complete the assessment and any support requirements.

By the end of the training sessions, each CMT had their own implementation plan specifying how the assessment would be completed and how action plans based on the assessment would be produced by the end of August 1999.

Following training, each CMT was provided with ongoing support by members of the project team. The nature and level of support varied according to CMT identified need and ranged from facilitated workshops to responding to minor queries as and when these arose. However, regular contact was maintained with all the CMTs during July and August, to ensure that the process of assessment was proceeding as planned and provide a reminder of the help/advice that could be accessed if required.

3.8 Learning points

All the CMTs successfully completed their baseline assessments and produced clear action plans based on their identified strengths and areas for improvement. The initial project review was carried out by the members of the Project Board, which included a CMT Programme Director and a Trust Associate Director with responsibility for four of the ten CMTs. Both of these individuals had been heavily involved in the implementation of the assessment by their particular CMTs. The Project Board review was also able to take account of views regarding the assessment process and tool that had actually been written on completed assessment documents, as well as comments that had been made to the Project Manager. The time-scale for development of the baseline assessment did not allow for thorough piloting of the tool prior to its use and it was decided that further project work should be undertaken within the Trust, in order to:

- More fully evaluate the baseline assessment tool through a focus group involving representatives from all the CMTs.
- Develop a revised tool to be used in future re-assessments.
- Ensure that the results of re-assessments are integrated closely within the Trust's business planning process.
- Identify and implement mechanisms for ongoing support to CMTs as they take an increasingly wider role within the organisational business planning process.

The review findings demonstrated that there had been some obvious process difficulties for the CMTs in completing their assessments:

- The tight time-scale to train the CMTs in the use of the tool and to complete the assessment had resulted in CMT members feeling 'under some degree of pressure'.
- There was variability between CMTs with regard to their ability to cover the depth of assessment required. This in part related to their level of maturity as teams, e.g., difficulties relating to CMT members' level of knowledge of what processes were actually in place across all service areas.
- As this was a new process, it required considerable time to complete (several hours' work from each CMT, and involving more than one session or meeting), and this led to practical difficulties getting the teams together to carry out the work.
- In some cases, where CMTs covered a wide range of discrete service areas, it was difficult to achieve a service-wide view. This meant that the team found itself carrying out a number of service-specific assessments, rather than a single "service-wide" assessment.

The review findings also identified problems relating to the design and content of the assessment tool itself as follows:

- The level of detail within the assessment tool could lead to CMTs becoming 'bogged down' in the detail and losing awareness of what the assessment was actually trying to achieve.

- Some CMT members felt that even more detailed training in the use of the Model would have been beneficial in giving a greater understanding of the Model and thus enabling a more informed assessment.
- Difficulties were more apparent with the Results Section than the Enablers Section. CMTs generally found it quite hard to identify appropriate measures across all the areas covered, although they were more familiar with understanding the approaches taken to ensuring quality. They had particular difficulties identifying trends, tended not to have set targets and were not on the whole engaged in either internal or external benchmarking. It was recognised that these were new areas of involvement for the CMTs, and this stimulated much debate. However, the point was also made that this raised CMT members' awareness of the role of performance monitoring within clinical governance and of the benefits of being more focused on outcomes/results.

Several positive features of the assessment tool and overall process were also identified:

- Although initially a little daunting due to the breadth of detail contained within the assessment, once started, the process was clear and completion became simpler as the CMTs progressed with the assessment
- The content was found to be relevant
- Coverage was comprehensive
- The assessment tool generated a lot of useful discussion within CMTs and provided an opportunity for the teams to explore in detail some of the current issues relating to their services
- It was described as an 'empowering' and constructive process by many people, which gave the CMTs some clear definition of their roles and responsibilities, enabled them to think objectively about their services, gave them control over action planning, enabled them to work as a team and was generally seen as a learning opportunity
- Those CMTs who carried out the assessment as a team found the process most beneficial
- The assessment process and the comprehensive nature of the tool enabled the production of well considered action plans
- The guidelines were generally thought to be useful
- The rating tables looking at overall level of achievement were found to be generally useful and teams reached reasonable consensus, but the general

view was that identification of strengths and areas for improvement was most useful and in practical terms, formed a natural step into the development of an action plan.

On the basis of this work, it was agreed that clinical governance assessment should become an annual process linked clearly with the Trust annual corporate self-assessment and business planning processes. A revised assessment tool was produced in Spring 2000 and a programme of training and continued support for the CMTs planned, to enable them to complete their first annual re-assessment in the Autumn of that year.

3.9 Final thoughts on self-assessment and clinical governance

The baseline assessment project can be seen to have benefited the Trust in several ways. The whole project has assisted the CMTs to gain strength, direction, and greater clarity of purpose. The CMTs have appreciated and accepted the principle of self-assessment with their ownership of the baseline assessment results assured through their active participation in the assessment process. The process of self-assessment carried out within CMTs has led to ownership of the action-plans at service level and a greater understanding of the concepts of 'excellence'. The Trust has also gained strength from the fact that the assessment aligns closely with the corporate assessment process and has helped to achieve consistency across service areas. CMT assessment will now form an integral component of the Trust's broader annual cycle of self-assessment and improvement. Year on year comparisons against the CMTs' detailed action plans will be facilitated by the continuing use of the assessment tool.

3.10 The Benefits of using the Excellence Model

Since we adopted the Model in 1995, initially for self-assessment, it has made its influence known in all kinds of ways. Below is a snapshot of how using the Model has not only changed what we do, but how it has changed the way we think about things.

3.11 Stakeholder focus

Our first experience of using the Model for self-assessment forced us to be much clearer about who our stakeholders were, and what the relationship was between us. By being clearer about this, we could then better balance their (sometimes conflicting) requirements, weigh their relative importance to what we wanted to achieve as an organisation, and plan accordingly. As an organisation within the NHS, the complex configuration of relationships sometimes meant that the same stakeholder group could play different roles at different times, (for example, General Practitioners can be viewed as both commissioners and suppliers of health services). The current government's emphasis on collaboration (in contrast with the previous administration's promotion of competition), is commensurate with the 1999 (revised) Excellence Model's added focus on the importance of *partnerships*. Our relationship with our stakeholders has therefore been revisited recently, to explore ways of furthering partnership developments. Our stakeholder 'map' is shown below:

Fig. 3 Our Stakeholders:

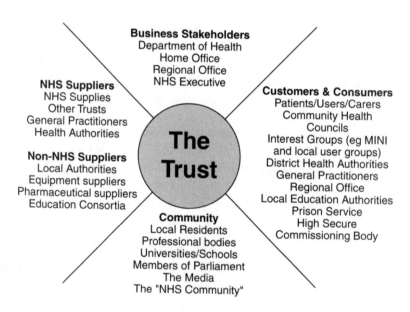

A key piece of work which commenced in June 2000, and is led by the Trust, within the context of the District's 'Health Action Zone' status, is a project to support the development of a 'new culture' of partnership working across public services within the District, using the Excellence Model. The project, *'Excellence Through Partnership'* aims to use the Model as a framework for assessing the current approach to joint working across the District, in order to enable the achievement of jointly agreed outcomes. The assessment process will enable the organisations involved to develop a more integrated and efficient approach to working together. Areas for continuous improvement will be identified and incorporated into the appropriate joint strategies and plans, (eg Health Improvement Plan and Health Action Zone plans) and recommendations will be made regarding a future 'best practice' approach to the integrated identification and delivery of Health Improvement Plan goals and outcomes.

3.12 Business Planning

The outcome of the annual organisational self-assessment and clinical governance self-assessments is now fully integrated into the Business Planning cycle, to help both prioritise action and ensure an effective review mechanism. The diagram below illustrates the role that self-assessment plays in the Business Planning process, which also involves working with, and seeking information from the various stakeholder groups identified above:

Fig. 4 Self-assessment and the Business Planning cycle

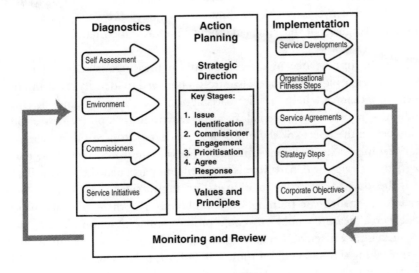

3.13 Trends, targets and comparisons

Our first self-assessment revealed some quite low scores in the 'Results' section. Although we considered ourselves to be 'results oriented' (one of the principles underpinning the Model), what the Model required us to have in place to demonstrate this found us wanting. This didn't necessarily mean that we weren't achieving good results. What it meant was that we didn't have the right measures, trends, targets, or comparisons in many relevant areas to demonstrate clearly:

- that we were achieving what we set out to achieve as detailed in our Policy and Strategy
- whether our performance was getting better, year on year, in some important areas
- how well our results compared with other organisations doing similar things.

What using the Model has helped us to do is to change the way we think about the performance measures that are important to us, and what we do with them. That is, the Model has not only helped refocus our attention on the need to set appropriate targets, identify trends, and establish suitable comparators, but it acts as a check that we actually use this information to inform, and if necessary change, how we do things (i.e. our approach, or, using the language of the Model and how we address the Enablers).

Whilst the importance of direct perception measures is reflected in the Model's weightings, the Model also stresses the need to identify those internal measures that can help predict satisfaction (i.e. 'lagging' and 'leading' indicators respectively). Internal measures may indicate a problem area some time before the effects of the problem are reflected in perception measures. For example, sickness absence measures (internal measures) may show that a particular service or department is experiencing particular difficulties. These may be due to excessive workloads, unsupportive management, poor leadership, inadequate training, or a combination of these. The alarm bells that such a measure would ring could prompt remedial action. Waiting until the next staff satisfaction survey results (perception measures) are available before taking action could, for some staff at least, be too late in the day. Self-assessment helped define our deficit in this area, and consequently additional measures have been introduced, analysed and targeted:

Example 1 - Customer Results: Perception Measures - Patient's Charter survey
Since the end-users of what we provide form one of our key 'stakeholder' groups, we now measure their perceptions of the services we deliver in a number of ways. A major way of gathering feedback from them is the Trust's annual Local Patient's Charter survey. This has been undertaken since 1995. There is a national requirement for NHS Trusts to monitor achievement against the Patient's Charter standards, and the survey questionnaire we use is designed to identify user and carer perceptions of how well the Trust is achieving the Charter standards. The results of the survey are used to inform the quality improvement process within clinical services. By tracking our performance against the standards over time, we can be reassured that the approaches we have in place in the 'Enabler' side of the Model are having the desired effect. Such data gives examples of how positive trends can be discerned for many results, and shows evidence of maintenance of good performance against our standards for others. The targets we have now set for these Patient's Charter Standards reflect the importance the Trust places on maintaining these high levels of achievement.

Supported by qualitative measures of user satisfaction, and service-specific surveys, the Trust is able to target improvement areas by using the trend data, and comparisons against target. The impetus to set targets, and to identify trends over time, has stemmed largely from the 'gaps' in evidence revealed by using the Model for self-assessment.

The perception measures are now supported by a range of 'indicator' measures, which help us to predict levels of user satisfaction.

Example 2 - Customer Results: Performance Indicators - Pressure Sores
Pressure sores are a major source of pain and discomfort for patients and can potentially lead to long term disability through amputation or, in extreme cases, can be life threatening. Complications following a pressure sore inevitably also involve additional costs to the NHS through the provision of wound dressings, surgical interventions, and the provision of artificial limbs or wheelchairs. By identifying those patients at risk and taking preventive measures, our District Nurses have been able to achieve and maintain their target of a 50 % reduction in the incidence of pressure sores for those "at risk" patients on their caseloads, as the graph below illustrates:

Fig. 5 District Nursing pressure sore management

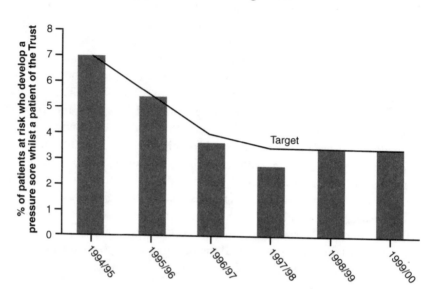

Example 3 - People Results: Perception measures - Staff Opinion Survey
Our first self-assessment against the Excellence Model identified a major 'area for improvement', that is, there was no systematic way of determining staff perceptions on a range of work-related issues considered to be important to them, so there was no data to trend or target. An annual staff opinion survey has been carried out since that time, designed to elicit staff perceptions to do with motivation and satisfaction. For example, the Trust invests significantly in the training and development of its staff, and needs to know how staff groups experience its approach across the Trust. In the annual survey, therefore, our staff are asked for their opinions on the training they receive in their job and their perception of the Trust's attitude towards training. The following figure shows examples of the responses to statements on this issue over the last four years.

Fig. 6 Examples of responses in the Staff Opinion Survey 1996 to 1999

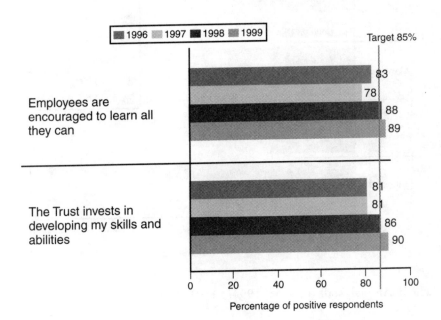

These overall responses are broken down into work areas, so that in those areas where achievement against targets is relatively low, or where trends are cause for concern, the responsible manager can then be helped to first of all determine the cause of the problem, and then take action (in the Enablers) to address it.

Example 4 - People Results: Performance Indicators - staff turnover
Prior to our first self-assessment, much data was routinely gathered for monitoring purposes without it being fully exploited as a 'leading' indicator of staff satisfaction. Our experience of using the Model has sharpened up the way we now use such data to inform our Human Resources strategy. For example, the overall turnover rates since the establishment of the Trust has reduced year on year, as shown in the following figure:

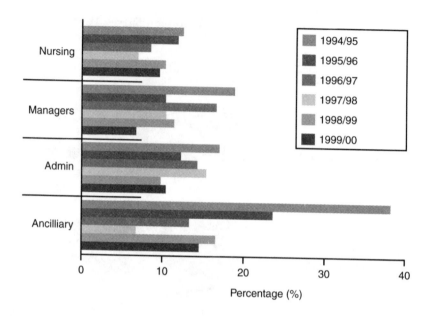

Fig. 7 Annual staff turnover, 1994/5 to 1999/00

Generally speaking a downward trend in staff turnover is seen as positive, indicating staff satisfaction and offering stability and continuity to patient care. As the data shows, turnover of all staff groups has improved over the past six years. In particular, there is a much-reduced turnover in ancillary and maintenance staff. This is a reflection of changes that were introduced in the form of multiskilling of our facilities personnel (i.e. a changed approach on the Enablers side of the Model) into ways of working, targeted at this group in particular to address the high turnover in the earlier years. Similarly, action taken in 1999, following the higher turnover rate recorded for nursing during 1998/99, had the desired effect of reducing the turnover rate during 1999/00. Staff turnover also provides an example of how the Trust has benchmarked some of its performance results against that of other organisations. Benchmarking against the Pay & Workforce Review (PWR) average for other NHS Trusts, for example, shows that the Trust's turnover is below average.

Example 5 - Key Performance Results: Performance Outcomes; Management Costs
In common with many NHS providers, we have been required to make considerable savings over recent years. Since April 1995, we have been subject to an additional financial target by the NHS Executive for the maximum spending on management costs, as part of the NHS objective to concentrate funds on direct patient care. This principle is integral to our values and business objectives. For example, a key outcome of the improvements to our computerised financial systems (changes to the Enabler 'Partnerships and Resources'), has been the reduction in manpower resources required to deliver the finance and payroll functions. In April 1993, we employed 33 whole time equivalent staff compared to 22 as at December 1998. In line with organisational policy and strategy, this rationalisation of staffing has been achieved through natural wastage.

Example 6 - Key Performance Results: Performance Indicators - 'Blocked Beds'
Like many similar Trusts, we have patients in our beds who have received treatment and are well enough to be discharged. However, the appropriate support in the community has still to be arranged. Whilst not discharging the patient avoids the possibility of them becoming a candidate for early readmission, the fact that a bed is being unnecessarily occupied means that another patient is potentially being denied access to an acute bed for which they may have an urgent need. The beds occupied by these patients are referred to as 'blocked beds'. A series of detailed audits of bed occupancy has revealed that the most frequently cited reason for blocked beds is a lack of a place to stay following discharge. By working in partnership with Social Services colleagues who have a statutory responsibility for the provision of accommodation, we have been able to improve this situation. Figure 8 shows that we have been successful in reducing the number of blocked beds from 716 in Sept 1997, to 549 in Sept 1999. The original target was to reduce this figure to 500 by Sept 2001, (later revised to 500 in 2000).

Fig. 8 Number of Blocked Beds for Sept 1997 to Sept 1999

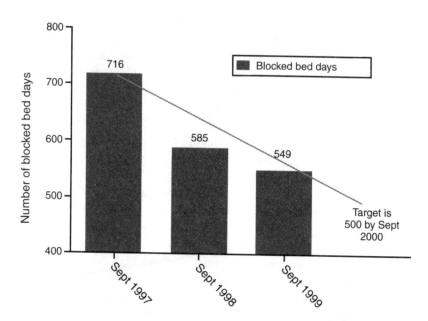

3.14   A clearer focus on improvement activities

Prior to adopting the Model, there was a good deal of activity already going on in the pursuit of continuous improvement. What using the Model has helped us achieve is a clearer focus on priorities for action. Each self-assessment results in a long list of potential 'areas for improvement', and it would be impossible (if not demotivating) to try and tackle them all. The Model encourages the setting of priorities in line with those things that the organisation deems important, and is made explicit in its vision and mission (found under the 'Leadership' section), or defined under 'Policy and Strategy'. Many of the identified improvement areas are addressed as discrete projects, and supported by our Quality, Evaluation and Development (QED) department. Areas that have been identified as priorities for action following the self-assessment, and in the context of relevance to the Business Plan, will then receive the appropriate level of support to ensure action.

3.15   Involving people in the process

Another benefit of using the Model has been in the way that it encourages the involvement of people at all levels across the Trust. As part of the self-assessment process, for instance, the assessment team interviews the Chief Executive and his Directors, and runs a number of focus groups that represent a wide cross section of staff. The interviews with the executive team are designed to both challenge and clarify. Directors are interviewed as members of a corporate team, with joint responsibility for issues, about areas on which they could bring specialist knowledge to bear. For example, interview questions might be along the lines of:

- *What has been done to address the key process issues identified following last year's self-assessment?*

- *What mechanisms are in place to ensure that the way we provide care is proven to be safe and effective?*

- *In what ways does the Trust show respect for people?*

- *How does the Trust encourage staff and patients to express their views?*

The staff focus groups are both single and multi-professional, and as much as possible we arrange to 'gatecrash' pre-existing groups that meet regularly, to minimise disruption to staff and avoid calling extraordinary meetings. A typical programme of focus groups includes community administrative staff, nurses, team leaders, HR staff, secretaries, child health staff, podiatrists etc. Within the staff focus groups, participants are encouraged to be open and honest about how they experience work-related issues. They may be asked questions such as:

- *Can you give examples of changes that have resulted from feedback you have given to your manager?*

- *Give examples of improvements to services that you have made as a result of feedback from customers.*

- *Tell us in what ways the Trust helps you to clearly understand your role and responsibilities.*

- *Can you give examples of where the Trust has fairly and consistently applied its employment policy and practices?*

The information obtained from the interviews and focus groups is used to supplement that obtained from the other sources (e.g. paper sources, staff opinion survey), helps to confirm the impact that approaches are having, and acts as a check on how widely they are being deployed.

The involvement of so many people from different organisational levels that using the Model has stimulated, has also reiterated the message that people's views are valued and welcomed, irrespective of their role and position.

3.16   A strategic and operational framework

Although the Model was used predominantly for self-assessment purposes following its introduction into the Trust, it soon became apparent that it had much more to offer. For example, the Excellence Model is now used to underpin the development of Policy and Strategy. In some cases, it is used as a framework, such as the Strategic Direction, Clinical Effectiveness Strategy, Quality and Clinical Governance Strategy and Nursing and Specialist Clinical Professions Strategy. In some cases it is used as well as a tool to identify further action required. The Model is also used to set definitive themes for our policy and planning stages, using a diagnostic, action planning, implementation and monitoring approach, as described above.

Through the wider use of the Model for purposes in addition to self-assessment, the Trust is now able to ensure more explicit alignment between Policy and Strategy and the actions of teams and individuals to support it. Directors' objectives, for example, are derived from the Annual Plan using the Model's criteria headings. Departmental heads and other managers are then able to plan their action, and that of their teams, in a way that supports the achievement of those objectives. Through the process of Quality Performance Management, all staff have annual objectives which support the achievement of Director objectives and which reflect the criteria of the Model. This ensures ultimately that all levels of the organisation have objectives that have a clear focus on what Policy and Strategy has stated is important for the Trust to achieve.

3.17   Personal benefits

It is worth noting at this point that for the members of the self-assessment team, a number of personal and professional benefits have been reported. These include:

Increased knowledge:
* Increased theoretical and practical knowledge about TQM principles and practices and the self-assessment process
* Detailed understanding of the organisation.

Skills development:
* Practical experience of teamworking, reporting and project management skills
* Opportunities to develop communication, negotiation and influencing skills
* Involvement in presentations and training sessions for other staff
* Advising on use of the model in the development of policy and strategy.

Continuing professional development:
* Opportunities to work with more senior colleagues
* Raised personal profile and visibility within the Trust
* Networking opportunities both inside and outside the Trust.

3.18   Introducing and sustaining the use of the Excellence Model - what helped?

There is no doubt that since adopting the Excellence Model in 1995, by carrying out regular self-assessments against it, and by using the framework as a structure for Strategies, and Clinical Governance, that it has been successfully integrated into the organisation in many ways. The fact that this is so has been aided in large measure by the existence of a number of factors.

3.19   A culture of continuous quality improvement

As evidenced by the WPCHT's 'Quality Journey', described at the beginning of this case study, there already existed a strong CQI culture within the Trust. Investors in People, and Charter Mark accreditation had already been achieved, and there was a history of staff involvement in a wide variety of smaller scale, quality improvement projects. The principles that underpin the Excellence Model - customer focus, people development and involvement, leadership and consistency of purpose, continuous improvement, and results orientation, for example - were principles already reflected in the dominant culture of the Trust at the time it was adopted by the organisation. Had this fertile ground not existed, it is unlikely that introducing the Model at the time would have been so well received and supported by the senior team.

As with many organisations though, the Trust was host to a number of sub-cultures, due at least in part to the fact that when the Trust was first established, it brought together two quite disparate organisations. Not everyone in the sub-cultures embraced the concepts of continuous improvement. What was important, though, was that the conducive culture permeated the senior ranks within the organisation. The very act of introducing the Model, demonstrating benefits, and involving more and more people as its use has become more widespread, has served to bring about cultural changes in those sub-cultures initially resistant to the continuous improvement ethos. In fact, some organisations introduce the model for the very purpose of bringing about a culture change. Our experience is that an enabling culture must already exist at the senior level at least, for the Model and its associated activities to get off the ground.

3.20 Commitment

Already referred to on several occasions earlier in the case study, this really has been so important that it bears revisiting. The decision to adopt and use the Excellence Model as a way of improving organisational effectiveness should not be undertaken lightly. It demands a great deal - in time, energy, resources - if real benefit is to be gained. Using the Model for self-assessment means that organisational flaws are identified and made explicit, work results from the need to address them, stamina is required to 'stick with it' when the going gets tough, and in some areas considerable effort may be expended with little evidence of improvement *in the short term*. All this takes commitment. In our case, it started with the Chief Executive and his senior team (also charged with driving the conducive culture referred to above) and has had to be evident in all those who have a role to play in translating the concepts of the Model into practical organisational benefit. Visible, active commitment to using the Model as a way of improving the effective management of the organisation, is probably the single most important factor that will determine whether or not the Model survives in its host organisation.

3.21 Acting on the results

Carrying out self-assessment against the Model will, in itself change nothing. It is a diagnostic tool and, as with other forms of diagnosis, needs follow-up, and remedial action. At WPCHT, there is, and has always been, what Peters and Waterman (1982) referred to as a 'bias for action'. The results of a self-assessment exercise may well be 'interesting', but will not lead to sustained change unless planned, prioritised actions result from it. The Trust uses a common project management framework to ensure that all such actions are appropriately planned, monitored and evaluated for effectiveness. Early experience of improvement projects that went off track, over timescale, and off focus, led to the realisation that equal rigour needed to be afforded to the ensuing improvement plans and activities as to the self-assessment process itself.

3.22 Co-ordination of improvement projects

The longer we have worked with the Excellence Model, the more we have come to recognise the importance of the linkages between various elements of it. Similarly, improvement activities that are indicated as a result of self-assessment often have linkages with other improvement activities identified by a different 'cluster' of 'areas for improvement'. What helps us to avoid unnecessary duplication and overlap is to ensure that the various improvement programmes are co-ordinated. Although many improvement projects are co-ordinated by the Trust's Quality, Evaluation and Development (QED) department, which has an overview of an annual programme of improvement projects for which it provides support, it also helps to have certain key individuals at senior level who are 'board members' on a number of projects to provide a similar co-ordinating and overview function.

3.23 Conclusion

The Excellence Model is used so extensively within the Trust now, that it is hard to imagine organisational life without it. In a host of ways, the use of the Model has become integral to the way we plan, deliver and review what we do. It is important to remember, though, that it is just a Model, a representation, and that it is there as a tool and not a master. As someone probably famous once said, '*All models are wrong - some are useful*'. Our experience has been that, as long as we use the Model in ways that make sense to us, and that fit with our own priorities, it is a highly useful model. In fact, it seems to us that the Model always makes sense - our decisions about the applicability of it have been mostly to do with relative relevance, rather than logic (e.g. over how much attention to focus on some of the 'areas to address' in the Model).

From the early days, when the Model was first used for a 'stand-alone' self-assessment to the present, which sees the full integration between self-assessment *and* clinical governance and the Business Planning cycle, and which sees the Model's framework being used to structure key strategic documents, significant strides have been taken. Some results are tangible - they can be analysed, targeted, and compared. Other results, though less tangible, are nevertheless significant. These are to do with how using the Model has influenced the way we think about what we do. In a sense, the Model throws down the gauntlet - using it can't help but challenge and sometimes it can be painful. The decision to adopt the Model was not taken lightly, and sticking with it has not come without considerable commitment and effort. But the rewards have certainly been there. We expect that greater rewards will be reaped as our experience of using the Model continues to mature.

References

Department of Health (1998). A First Class Service. London: HMSO

Department of Health (1999). Clinical Governance: Quality in the new NHS. London: HMSO

Hakes, C. and Reed, D. (1997). Organisational self-assessment for public sector excellence. Bristol: Bristol Quality Centre Ltd.

Peters, T. J. & Waterman, R.H. (1982) In Search of Excellence. Harper & Row. New York

Bibliography

British Quality Foundation: *Guide to the Business Excellence Model: Defining World Class*; (1998)

Crumley, H & Black, S. *Excellence in action*. Total Quality Management, July 1998, Vol., Issue 4/5, pS41-S45.

Department of Health. *The New NHS: Modern, dependable*. (1997).The Stationery Office.

Eskildsen, J.K & Kanji G.K. *Identifying the vital few using the EFQM Model*. Total Quality Management, July 1998, Vol. 9, Issue 4/5, S92-S95.

Eskildsen, J.K, Dahlgaard, J.J & Norgaard, A: *The impact of creativity and learning on business Excellence*. Total Quality Management., July 1999, Vol. 10; Issue 4,523-530.

Health Manpower Mgt. *Using Business Excellence model to effectively manage change within clinical support services*: Health Manpower Management 4/1/98, Vol. 24 (Number 2), 76-81.

Mann, R. *Business Excellence. Does self assessment work?* Food Manufacture, July 1998. Vol.73, 33-35.

Martensen, A & Dahlgaard, J: *Integrating business excellence and innovation management; developing vision, blueprint and strategy for innovation in creative and learning organisations*. Total Quality Management, July 1999, Vol.10, Issue 4/7, 627-636.

Russell, S: *Business excellence: from outside in or inside out?* Total Quality Management, July 1999, Vol. 10; Issue 4/5; 647-653.

Schon, D.A. *The reflective practitioner*; New York.Basic Books. 1983

Index

Just in time, 12

Key customer facing processes, 43,49
key lessons, 71
Key Performance Results, 22,
54,91,95,103,147
key support processes, 47, 49
key to success, 106

Lagging, 142
Leadership, 14, 19, 23,31, 44,
83,87,90,91
    issues, 23
    team strength, 37
Leadership development, 80,102
Leadership Effectiveness Analysis, 77,90
Leadership project, 76,78,79,80
Leicester Royal Infirmary, 83
lessons learnt, 107
level of information, 28
Likert scale, 91
Line management structure, 118
local self assessment, 27,39

Malcolm Baldrige Quality Award,
17,113,114
management domains, 5
management processes, 12
management systems, 5
managing risks, 35
Mayo Clinic, 17
medical services, 47
Model criterion parts, 48

National Plan, 105
National Service Framework, 89
National Specialist Learning Centre, 105
NHS 3, 66,67,90,147
NHS Executive, 15
non-clinical quality, 9
Northern & Yorkshire NHSE, 106

NVQ, 103
Organisational effectiveness, 122
organisational development, 105
organisational Learning, 4
organisational results, 25
Our Journey to Excellence, 75
outputs/outcomes, 89

Pareto charts, 28
Partnerships & Resources, 147
partnerships, 140
Patient Administrative System, 92
Patient Centred Care, 67,69
Patient Charter Standards, 16,143
Patient Charter survey, 133,143
Patient Perception Group, 66
patient survey method, 91,
Pay & Workforce Review, 146
PCGs, 112,
PCTs, 112
people management, 102, 122
people results, 144, 145
people satisfaction, 121
person specifications, 31
performance framework, 89
performance indicators, 28
performance management, 30,88,90
    - system, ,37,39
    -review, 51
performance monitoring, 51
PFI, 65
policy & strategy, 23, 44, 102,
103,132,148
primary and secondary care, 13
process centred organisation, 83
process performance framework, 89
process leaders, 90
process redesign stages, 84, 87,102
processes, 22
Project Board, 136
pursuit of Excellence, 3

Putting People First, 66

QDT, 12,
QED, 148, 153
Quality Award, 18
Quality Circle, 67
quality cycle, 4
Quality Development Teams, 9, 12,30,31
quality development, 4
quality improvement models, 113
quality management, 4
      -activities, 6
      -clinical & non-clinical, 11
quality state, 6
quality tools , 1,2
quality: definitions, 6

RADAR logic, 45,46
rating table, 135
redesign, 83, 84
Reflection on practice, 2
Resource Management Initiative, 3,4
Resources, 22
results, 43
reward & recognition, 81,82
rewards of model, 154
role of facilitation, 31
roles of key managers, 51- 52

Salford Royal Hospital NHS Trust, 1-3, 7
Schon, 2
self assessment, 2,12,
17,20,27,32,33,41,51,56,58,69
    114,115,117,118,128,148
    -baseline score, 15
    -organisational, 15
    -methods, 16,21,42,
    73,116,130,138
    -proforma, 18,19,21,21,28,35,
    -criteria, 21,24
    -local, 27,39

    -corporate, 27, 51, 73, 91, 105,
    116, 133
    -review framework, 53
    -team, 56,57
    -benefits, 69,139
    -South Tees approach, 70
    -reasons for, 73,129
    -stages of: 115,122-123,131,141
    -learning points, 123
Self Managed Trusts, 7
self motivation, 30
Service of Agreements, 35
set of indicators, 25
sharing good practice, 84
sources of information, 117
South Cleveland Hospitals, 105
South Tees Acute Hospitals, 63,65
staff opinion surveys, 144
staff surveys, 92
staff turnover, 145
STAHT core values, 77
storyboard format, 18
Strategic & Business plans, 28
strategy development, 18
strengths/areas for improvement, 35
sub-process diagram, 122
successes attained, 58
survey administration, 94
survey response rate, 123
sustainable continuous improvement, 14

Teamscore, 72
top down-bottom up systems, 5
TQM approach, 11
TQM, 3,4, 58,59,66,113
training programme & strategy, 19
Trust Standing Financial Instructions, 51
Trust Board Management Group, 65,66
Trust Board Quarterly Award, 30
Trust quality management approach, 30